# CYSTIC FIBROSIS

# MOLECULAR MEDICINE

*Advisory editors*

K. E. DAVIES, T. FRIEDMANN, P. GOODFELLOW
G. STAMATOYANNOPOULOS, D. J. WEATHERALL

P. Goodfellow (ed.): *Cystic fibrosis*
K. E. Davies (ed.): *The fragile X syndrome*

# Cystic Fibrosis

Edited by
PETER GOODFELLOW
*Imperial Cancer Research Fund Laboratories,
London*

Oxford   New York   Tokyo
OXFORD UNIVERSITY PRESS
1989

Oxford University Press, Walton Street, Oxford OX2 6DP
Oxford New York Toronto
Delhi Bombay Calcutta Madras Karachi
Petaling Jaya Singapore Hong Kong Tokyo
Nairobi Dar es Salaam Cape Town
Melbourne Auckland
and associated companies in
Berlin Ibadan

Oxford is a trade mark of Oxford University Press

© Oxford University Press and the contributors listed on p. ix, 1989

All rights reserved. No part of this publication may be reproduced, stored in a retrieval system, or transmitted, in any form or by any means, electronic, mechanical, photocopying, recording, or otherwise, without the prior permission of Oxford University Press

This book is sold subject to the condition that it shall not, by way of trade or otherwise, be lent, re-sold, hired out, or otherwise circulated without the publisher's prior consent in any form of binding or cover other than that in which it is published and without a similar condition including this condition being imposed on the subsequent purchaser

British Library Cataloguing in Publication Data
Cystic fibrosis.
1. Man. Pancreas. Cystic fibrosis
I. Goodfellow, P. (Peter), 1951-    II. Series
616.3'7
ISBN 0-19-261835-0

Library of Congress Cataloging-in-Publication Data
Cystic fibrosis/edited by Peter Goodfellow
(Molecular medicine)
Includes bibliographies.
1. Cystic fibrosis. I. Goodfellow, P. (Peter), 1951-
II. Series: Molecular medicine (Oxford, England)
[DNLM: 1. Cystic Fibrosis. WI 820 C996541]
RC858.C95C93 1989   616.3'7—dc 19   88-36931
ISBN 0-19-261835-0 (pbk.)

Set by Colset Private Limited
Printed in Great Britain by
J.W. Arrowsmith Ltd, Bristol

# Preface

Cystic fibrosis is a devastating genetic disease. Afflicted individuals can expect a drastically reduced quality of life and a curtailed lifespan. There is no such thing as a typical cystic fibrosis patient as each suffers from an overlapping combination of diverse symptoms. Nevertheless, the underlying defect is the same in all patients and current research implicates a defect in regulation of ion transport in secretory epithelia. Probably the most serious consequence of this defect is the production of abnormal, thick mucus which blocks the airways and promotes lung infection. Chronic infection results in gradual destruction of the lungs and this is a frequent cause of death. Advances in nutrition, physiotherapy, and antibiotic therapy have led to improvements in treatment; however, none of these approaches a cure. Strategies aimed at finding a cure need to be based on a better understanding of the fundamental defect and this will almost certainly require cloning the defective gene.

Everyone knows a carrier for the cystic fibrosis gene: in Caucasian populations one in every 20 individuals is a carrier. If two carriers marry and have children, on average, one in every four of their children will have this disease. This mode of inheritance is known as autosomal recessive and because carriers cannot be definitely recognized we all play Russian roulette when we have children. Recent advances have provided genetic markers that can be used for prenatal diagnosis in families in which an afflicted child has already been born. However, avoidance of the birth of afflicted children will require carrier testing the whole population and this will almost certainly require cloning the defective gene.

This book is designed to stimulate research at the interface between the medical and scientific professions. For the scientist interested in cystic fibrosis there is a description of the natural history, treatment, and prenatal diagnosis of the disease. For the clinician, there is a description of current research into the physiology and genetics of cystic fibrosis. Finding the basic defect and cloning the cystic fibrosis gene will be major advances. Converting those advances into clinical practice will require continued collaboration between the basic sciences and medicine.

Finally, I would like to pay tribute to the Cystic Fibrosis Research Trust. This charity is a reflection of the faith of families with cystic fibrosis that basic and clinical research can offer hope for cure and eradication of this terrible disease. This book is dedicated to that faith.

*London*
November 1988

P.N.G.

# Contents

| | | |
|---|---|---|
| | List of contributors | ix |
| **1** | **The natural history of cystic fibrosis** | **1** |
| | A.D.M. JACKSON | |
| | Introduction | 1 |
| | Genetics | 2 |
| | Pathogenesis | 2 |
| | Clinical features | 3 |
| | Diagnosis | 7 |
| | Family problems | 7 |
| | Problems in adolescence | 8 |
| | Prognosis | 8 |
| | References | 10 |
| **2** | **Management of cystic fibrosis** | **12** |
| | J.A. DODGE | |
| | Introduction | 12 |
| | The sweat abnormality | 13 |
| | Pancreatic insufficiency | 13 |
| | Nutritional problems | 14 |
| | Bowel complications | 15 |
| | Liver disease | 16 |
| | Respiratory disease | 17 |
| | Psychological problems | 20 |
| | Delivery of health care | 21 |
| | References | 22 |
| **3** | **Defects in epithelial ion transport in cystic fibrosis** | **24** |
| | A.W. CUTHBERT | |
| | Introduction | 24 |
| | Basic transepithelial transport processes | 24 |

viii    Contents

|   |   |
|---|---|
| Transport abnormalities in cystic fibrosis | 27 |
| Other systems | 34 |
| Other cell types | 34 |
| Other hypotheses | 36 |
| New approaches | 36 |
| Unknowns | 36 |
| Opportunities for therapeutic strategies | 37 |
| Note added in proof | 37 |
| References | 37 |

**4  Molecular genetics**  41
V. VAN HEYNINGEN AND D.J. PORTEOUS

|   |   |
|---|---|
| The molecular approach to genetic disease | 41 |
| Family studies | 42 |
| Classical genetics and assessement of candidate genes | 44 |
| Reverse genetics | 47 |
| Reverse genetics and the new technologies | 52 |
| References | 61 |

**5  Prenatal diagnosis**  66
D.J.H. BROCK

|   |   |
|---|---|
| Introduction | 66 |
| The risk of having a child with cystic fibrosis | 66 |
| DNA-based methods of prenatal diagnosis | 67 |
| Prenatal diagnosis of cystic fibrosis by linkage analysis | 70 |
| Microvillar enzyme-based prenatal diagnosis | 77 |
| Combining DNA and microvillar-based diagnosis | 85 |
| Summary | 86 |
| Addendum | 86 |
| References | 89 |

**Index**  93

# Contributors

D.J.H. BROCK  *Human Genetics Unit, University of Edinburgh, Western General Hospital, Edinburgh, EH4 2XU, UK.*

A.W. CUTHBERT  *Department of Pharmacology, University of Cambridge Medical School, Hills Road, Cambridge, CB2 2QD, UK.*

J.A. DODGE  *Institute of Clinical Science, The Queen's University of Belfast, Grosvenor Road, Belfast, BT12 6BJ, UK.*

V. VAN HEYNINGEN  *MRC Human Genetics Unit, Western General Hospital, Crewe Road, Edinburgh, EH4 2XU, UK.*

A.D.M. JACKSON  *Cystic Fibrosis Research Trust, 5 Blyth Road, Bromley, Kent, BR1 3RS, UK.*

D.J. PORTEOUS  *MRC Human Genetics Unit, Western General Hospital, Crewe Road, Edinburgh, EH4 2XU, UK.*

# 1 The natural history of cystic fibrosis

A.D.M. JACKSON

## Introduction

Cystic fibrosis (CF) is an inherited disease characterized by abnormal secretions of the exocrine glands. The abnormal secretions result in a variety of secondary clinical effects, including chronic lung disease and pancreatic insufficiency.

Although there had been several earlier reports of cases with the features of CF, the disease was first recognized as an entity by Fanconi *et al.* (1936) in a paper entitled 'The coeliac syndrome with congenital cystic pancreatic fibromatosis and bronchiectasis'. Dorothy Andersen (1938), a pathologist at the Babies Hospital in New York, gave the first detailed description of the clinical features and pathology of CF and called it 'Cystic fibrosis of the pancreas'. The cases she studied fell into three groups: a small group of babies who had died of neonatal obstruction, a larger group of children with chronic diarrhoea who had died of bronchopneumonia in the first few months of life, and another large group of older children who had died of chronic lung disease. Recognizing the role of sticky mucus as a cause of many of the symptoms, Farber (1945) invented the name 'mucoviscidosis' which became popular in North America for a time and is still used in France (*la mucoviscidose*). Andersen (1949) subsequently changed the name she had originally used to 'fibrocystic disease of the pancreas' and this term was used in English-speaking countries for some years. However, 'cystic fibrosis of the pancreas' gradually became the most popular name for the disease until it was shortened in the 1960s to 'cystic fibrosis', the name most frequently used today.

The pioneers in the clinical study of CF were Andersen and di Sant' Agnesi in New York; Fanconi and Rossi in Switzerland; Shwachman in Boston; and Bodian, Norman, and Young in London. These pioneers set up special CF clinics, carried out detailed clinical studies, and formulated management programmes. It was the New York group that first recognized the complication of acute salt loss caused by excessive sweating when it occurred in babies with CF during a heat-wave in the city in 1948 (Kessler and Andersen 1951). They subsequently demonstrated abnormally high salt levels in the sweat and saliva of CF patients and developed the diagnostic sweat test (di Sant' Agnesi *et al.* 1953).

In spite of detailed clinical investigation and intensive laboratory research in the past 50 years, CF remains an enigma. Nevertheless, progress has been made. The outlook for sufferers and their families has been transformed (Chapters 2 and 5), the mutant gene has been located precisely (Chapter 4), and we are close to a working hypothesis that might explain how the basic defect causes its widespread effects (Chapter 3).

## Genetics

The mutant gene, which has recently been located on the long arm of chromosome 7 (Knowlton *et al.* 1985; Wainwright *et al.* 1985; White *et al.* 1985), is transmitted as an autosomal recessive.

Cystic fibrosis is the commonest autosomal genetic disorder in populations of Caucasian origin, among whom the carrier rate is about 1 in 20 and the incidence about 1 in 2000 live births. The disease is much less common in African and Oriental races. In the United Kingdom there are about 5000 individuals with CF and over 300 affected babies are born annually. Because of the high carrier rate it has been postulated that there is a biological advantage in being a carrier but this has yet to be proved.

## Pathogenesis

The nature of the basic defect is not yet understood, but recent work has shown that there is defective transport of chloride ions across the lining epithelium of the nasal cavity and lower airways (Knowles *et al.* 1983*a*, 1983*b*) and of the sweat ducts (Quinton and Bijman 1983). These findings suggest a number of possible unifying hypotheses for the underlying pathophysiology of CF (Chapter 4).

Exocrine glands discharge their secretions either through ducts into body cavities or directly to various body surfaces, whereas endocrine glands secrete into the bloodstream. Most of the varied and widespread clinical manifestations of CF are due to the production of abnormal secretions by the exocrine glands. In the pancreas thick, semi-solid secretions obstruct the duct system from an early age so that the delivery of enzymes to the duodenum is considerably reduced. Deficiency of these enzymes impairs digestion and absorption, giving rise to nutritional deficiency. The glands lining the bowel wall secrete excessive amounts of viscid mucus which contribute to the malabsorption. Back-pressure in the pancreas from obstruction of the main ducts produces cysts and fibrosis in the body of the gland. The endocrine portion of the pancreas (islets of Langerhans) is usually unaffected by these structural changes in the rest of the gland, but the production of insulin is eventually reduced in some older patients.

In the liver similar obstruction of the bile ductules may result in cirrhosis and lead to back-pressure in the portal vein (portal hypertension). Total obstruction of the cystic duct may occur and this is associated with hypoplasia of the gall-bladder and the formation of gallstones.

The lungs are normal at birth but are prone to infection which stimulates the secretion of profuse amounts of sticky mucus. This causes obstruction, predisposing to further infection and secondary lung damage which in due course becomes irreversible.

The sweat glands are structurally normal but secrete abnormally high concentrations of sodium and chloride, the measurement of which forms the basis for the diagnostic sweat test (see below). In the salivary glands the changes are mainly functional, with abnormal concentrations of electrolytes, enzymes and other proteins, especially in the parotid.

The testes are normal but abnormalities of the vas deferens and epididymis, probably due to obstruction, render males sterile.

## Clinical features

Cystic fibrosis is present at birth, and in about 10 per cent of cases the diagnosis is made by sweat test a few weeks after birth and before symptoms develop, either because a previous child in the family is known to have the disease or as a result of a screening programme. A further 15 per cent of affected babies present immediately after birth with intestinal obstruction (meconium ileus). The majority of cases, however, present later in the first year with recurrent respiratory infections, diarrhoea, and failure to gain weight adequately (Table 1.1). Excluding babies with meconium ileus, the diagnosis is made before the age of one year in only about half the cases (Table 1.2) so it seems likely that many infants with typical symptoms are missed at this time. However, this is a disease which varies in severity and some patients have the disease in a mild form which is difficult to recognize

**Table 1.1.** Presenting features (approximate figures taken from various sources)

| | |
|---|---|
| Meconium ileus | 15% |
| Respiratory | 25% |
| Intestinal | 30% |
| Respiratory and intestinal | 15% |
| Family history | 10% |
| Others | 5% |

Table 1.2. Age at diagnosis, excluding meconium ileus (approximate figures taken from various sources)

| | |
|---|---|
| Under 6 months | 30% |
| 6 months to 1 year | 20% |
| 1–2 years | 20% |
| 2–5 years | 25% |
| Over 5 years | 5% |

until much later, even well into adult life. In one selected series of 65 adult patients 12 had been diagnosed after the age of 16 (Shwachman *et al.* 1965).

## Meconium ileus

The intestinal obstruction in babies with meconium ileus is caused by abnormally solid contents of the small bowel which have the consistency of putty. The baby fails to pass meconium after birth and shows increasing abdominal distension with bile-stained vomiting. The obstruction sometimes leads to perforation of the gut and secondary peritonitis. Abdominal X-rays show distended loops of bowel with fluid levels and a generalized opacity due to the abnormal meconium.

'Meconium ileus equivalent' is the inappropriate name given to a similar form of intestinal obstruction seen in some patients outside the neonatal period. 'Distal intestinal obstruction syndrome' is a cumbersome, if more accurate, alternative. The obstruction may be partial or complete and is often recurrent. The patient complains of abdominal pain and a soft mass can be felt in the abdomen. This complication has been reported in as many as 30 per cent of patients.

## Pancreatic insufficiency

Deficiency of pancreatic secretions gives rise to overt symptoms in most cases and is present to some degree in almost all. It results in abdominal distension and the passage of loose, bulky, fatty stools (steatorrhoea) which have a characteristic offensive smell. Babies fail to gain weight adequately in spite of a good appetite, but older patients may have poor appetites which contribute to the under-nourishment caused by malabsorption. Persistent diarrhoea may result in rectal prolapse and this can be the presenting feature.

## The respiratory tract

Both upper and lower respiratory tracts are affected. In the upper tract recurrent infection leads to thickening and hypertrophy of the mucous membranes of the nose and nasal sinuses with upper airway obstruction and in many cases polyp formation. Recurrent infections of the lower respiratory tract are the major cause of morbidity and mortality in CF. Starting early in life as acute obstructive bronchitis, these infections recur over a number of years and lead ultimately to irreversible lung damage. The profuse secretion of viscid mucus in response to infection easily obstructs the small peripheral airways in babies, causing a wheezy cough, indrawing of the soft parts of the chest wall, and overinflation of the lungs. There may be severe attacks of coughing associated with vomiting, suggesting the diagnosis of whooping cough.

As the child gets older, the infection becomes chronic and causes progressive damage to the lung structure. The cough and wheezing become persistent and there is copious purulent sputum. In advanced stages of the pulmonary disease the chest becomes barrel shaped due to chronic overinflation, the fingers are clubbed, and the patient blue and breathless. Blood may be coughed up (haemoptysis) and air may escape into the chest cavity following rupture of distended lung tissue (pneumothorax). As more and more lung tissue is damaged, back-pressure begins to build up in the right side of the heart. Finally, death results from a combination of respiratory and cardiac failure.

Fortunately, treatment now considerably modifies the natural history of lung disease in CF so that lung damage can be limited or delayed for many years, and most affected children lead an active school life. However, only those with the very mildest form of the disease escape lung involvement entirely.

The causal agents of respiratory infections in CF are both viral and bacterial. Viral infections frequently start in the upper respiratory tract and descend to cause bronchitis. Measles and influenza viruses are particularly likely to cause lower respiratory infections in patients with CF. The commonest bacterial organisms infecting the lungs in young children are *Staphylococcus aureus* and *Haemophilus influenzae*. In older patients with purulent sputum *Pseudomonas aeruginosa* is almost always present in the respiratory tract but not necessarily as a pathogen. Some patients show an allergic reaction in the lungs to the fungus *Aspergillus fumigatus*, with a positive skin test and changes in the lung X-ray which disappear rapidly with treatment.

The typical X-ray appearances in the lungs of CF patients are: thickening of the peripheral bronchial walls, hyperinflation, small opacities in the lung fields due to patches of collapse or consolidation, and enlarged hilar glands. In advanced cases there are segmental areas of collapse and widespread dense patchy shadows indicating abscesses. Lung function tests reflect the degree of pulmonary pathology.

## The liver

Focal biliary cirrhosis is clinically evident in about 10 per cent of older patients although it is present to some degree in many more, as indicated by autopsy findings. Liver function tests become abnormal before enlargement of the liver can be detected clinically. The complication of portal hypertension causes enlargement of the spleen and may result in the vomiting of blood from dilated veins in the oesophagus (haematemesis). The progress of liver disease in CF is variable but is usually slow and sub-clinical. However, a few patients do go on to develop liver failure with fluid in the abdominal cavity (ascites).

## Growth and nutrition

The mean birth weight of babies with CF is about 5 per cent lower than that of normal babies. Subsequent growth depends on the severity of the pulmonary disease, the frequency of respiratory infections, the degree of malabsorption, and the extent to which treatment modifies these conditions. Thirty years ago less than 10 per cent of affected children were above the normal 25th centile for height and weight, but nowadays steady increases in both height and weight can be expected in the first 10 years of life, although the medians run roughly along the 25th centile. There is a falling off of growth between the ages of 10 and 15 which is more marked in weight than in height. Puberty and skeletal maturity are usually delayed, so that growth in height continues for a longer period than normal and the median mature height falls well above the 10th centile. Final heights and weights are greater in those who have been relatively free of respiratory symptoms, and there is marked stunting of growth and wasting in those with a long history of lung disease.

## Diabetes

The complication of diabetes occurs in about 10 per cent of older patients with CF, and is usually mild. It can mostly be controlled with oral drugs, and complications are rare.

## Arthropathy

A characteristic form of joint disease (arthropathy) occurs in a small number of adolescents and adults with CF. The onset is usually acute with painful swollen joints and fever. The attack settles down after a week or so but often recurs. The joints most often affected are the knees and ankles. The cause of this episodic arthropathy is not clear. Hypertrophic pulmonary osteo-arthropathy, a condition in which the bones are affected as well as the joints, has also been reported in adults with CF, and is related to acute exacerbations of respiratory infection.

## Diagnosis

The diagnosis of CF is established by finding a raised level of sodium and chloride in the sweat of patients with a suggestive clinical picture. The standard method for the sweat test is the technique of pilocarpine iontophoresis first described by Gibson and Cooke (1959). Sweating is induced by passing a tiny electrical current into the skin of the forearm through a filter paper soaked in a solution of pilocarpine. The skin is then dried and cleaned and sweat is collected for 30 minutes. The weight of sweat and its sodium and chloride content are measured. At least 100 mg of sweat is needed for a reliable result. In such a serious disease the accuracy of the one diagnostic test is obviously crucial and can only be guaranteed if the test is done by someone who is experienced and is performing the test regularly. It is not uncommon for mistakes in diagnosis to occur and these are usually due to inadequate performance of the sweat test.

It is difficult to obtain enough sweat for the standard sweat test from babies in the first few weeks of life, and measurement of immunoreactive trypsin (IRT) in the blood has been developed as a neonatal screening test. This test is based on the fact that affected babies have a leak-back of pancreatic trypsin into the blood from the obstructed pancreas. The IRT test can be done on the dried blood spot that is obtained from all babies on the 7th to 10th day of life for screening for phenylketonuria and hypothyroidism. Babies with positive IRT tests must have the investigation repeated at two weeks, by which time the number of false results is very small. By reason of its high selectivity and specificity, the IRT test is the most reliable test for CF screening in the new-born (Kuzemko 1986). No decision has yet been taken to embark on screening for CF on a national basis in the United Kingdom.

In almost all cases of CF there is some evidence of malabsorption or pancreatic deficiency. This can be demonstrated by finding an excess of fat on microscopy of the stools, or an excretion of more than 5 g of fat per day over a three-day period on a normal fat intake. It may occasionally be necessary to use more sophisticated tests of pancreatic function when the diagnosis of pancreatic deficiency remains in doubt.

## Family problems

Although CF is no longer a cause of death in early childhood, that possibility hangs over a family like the Sword of Damocles. Cystic fibrosis, like most chronic diseases of childhood, is a family problem and in the early days after the diagnosis has been made the burden falls heavily on the parents. It may take years for them to come to terms with the problems of a chronic progressive disease. Anxiety for the child's future coupled with immediate practical problems, such as frequent hospital visits and organizing daily routines for physiotherapy and medication, cause stress in most families, to the point of breakdown in some. Depression and other nervous problems are commoner in families with a CF child than in the population as a whole, the mothers being more often affected than the fathers. The knowledge that they are carriers of a genetic disease inevitably causes parents to feel guilty and to worry about the possibility that future children may inherit the disease. For the affected children, the gradual realization that they are different from their healthy companions and siblings and that they are at risk from premature death is a potential source of emotional disturbance. There are additional emotional problems for the survivor if one of two affected siblings dies. In spite of this, most CF children and their families now cope surprisingly well with their problems, encouraged no doubt by the improved outlook.

## Problems in adolescence

The normal stresses of adolescence are increased by having a chronic, incurable, and life-threatening disease. This is also a time when the stressful change of consultant from paediatrician to adult physician is likely to take place. Delayed sexual and limited physical development can affect relationships with the opposite sex. Boys have to bear the knowledge that they are sterile and young women have to accept that pregnancy must be avoided if their clinical state is not good.

Social life has its problems. Treatment programmes are demanding, and the cough is socially embarrassing. Regular daily physiotherapy may be difficult to arrange and interferes with the normal routine. Some adolescents rebel against this obtrusion of treatment into their lives and refuse to cooperate with their physician. For those who have frequent lower respiratory infections, attendance at school or work may be interrupted by admissions to hospital. Adjusting to independent living after so many years of dependence on parents may be difficult. Nevertheless, most adolescents with CF have learnt to cope with adversity and can overcome these difficulties.

## Prognosis

The prognosis for patients with CF has steadily improved over the past 50 years, and there are three main reasons for this. First, the advent of antibiotics in the early 1940s; secondly, the improvement in other methods of treatment; and thirdly, the more frequent recognition of mild cases and their inclusion in the survival figures. It is also widely believed that the trend towards earlier diagnosis, and hence the earlier commencement of treatment, improves prognosis. Clinical experience supports this belief, although it has not been proved by controlled investigation.

**Table 1.3.** Survival rates

| Series | Survival to age | |
|---|---|---|
| | 10 years | 20 years |
| All USA, 1966[1] | 24% | |
| USA, CF centres, 1966[1] | | 25% |
| USA, CF centres, 1982[2] | | 50% |
| Denmark, non-centres, 1945–1981[3] | 52% | |
| Denmark, CF centres, 1945–1981[3] | 84% | 61% |
| All England and Wales, 1980[4] | 77% | 62% |
| Melbourne, Australia, CF centre, 1980[4] | 91% | 80% |

[1]Warwick and Pogue (1969); [2]Warwick (1982); [3]Nielsen and Schiotz (1982); [4]Phelan and Hey (1984).

Before 1939 the majority of patients died in the first year of life, but survival rates have improved enormously since then. It has also become clear that centres of excellence in the management of CF have significantly better results than the average. Table 1.3 shows the improvement in survival to the ages of 10 and 20 years in various series of patients, and the difference in survival rates between patients who attend CF centres and those who do not. According to Warwick (1982) the survival rates for CF centres are at least five times better than those for non-centres. In England and Wales, as a whole, 80 per cent of affected infants survive to the age of 9 years, whereas in the Victoria State special CF centre in Melbourne, Australia 80 per cent survive to the age of 20 (Phelan and Hey 1984). For some 200 patients over the age of 16 attending the special CF clinic at the Brompton Hospital, London from 1965 to 1980 there was a 25 per cent chance of surviving to the age of 30 years (Duncan *et al.* 1981). In most surveys, the survival rate is slightly higher for boys than for girls, although the reason for this has not been explained. Most reports also indicate a higher than average mortality among patients who present with meconium ileus but, if surgical treatment is successful and early respiratory infections are aggressively treated, there need be no long-term disadvantage for babies with meconium ileus (Mearns 1969).

Not only are large numbers of patients surviving to adult life, but their quality of life is improving. In 1976 in Boston, USA, there were 70 patients over the age of 25, of whom the oldest was 44. The majority had no serious disability and were employed in a wide range of occupations, and six of the women had borne children (Shwachman *et al.* 1976). At the Brompton Hospital almost 90 per cent of 183 adolescent or adult patients attending in 1982 were in full-time education or employment and only three were too ill to work (Batten 1983).

These data for life expectancy and the quality of life relate to patients who were first treated between 10 and 20 years ago. In view of the considerable advances in treatment since then, it seems likely that the child who is diagnosed today can expect to survive well into adult life without severe lung disease and with a greatly improved quality of life.

## References

Andersen, D. H. (1938). Cystic fibrosis of the pancreas and its relation to celiac disease: a clinical and pathological study. *American Journal of Diseases of Children* **56**, 344–99.

Andersen, D. H. (1949). Therapy and prognosis of fibrocystic disease of the pancreas. *Pediatrics* **3**, 406–18.

Batten, J. C. (1983). The adolescent and adult. In *Cystic fibrosis*, (ed. M. E. Hodson, A. P. Norman and J. C. Batten), pp. 209. Ballière Tindall, London.

Duncan, F. R., Hodson, M. E., and Batten J. C., (1981). Cystic fibrosis—survival into adult life. *European Journal of Paediatrics* **137**, 125.

Fanconi, G., Uehlinger, E., and Knauer, C. (1936). The coeliac syndrome with congenital cystic pancreatic fibromatosis and bronchiectasis. *Wiener Medizinischer Wochenschrift* **86**, 753–6.

Farber, S. (1945). Some organic digestive disturbances in early life. *Journal of the Michigan State Medical Society* **44**, 406–18.

Gibson, L. E. and Cooke, R. E. (1959). A test for concentration of electrolytes in sweat in cystic fibrosis of the pancreas utilizing pilocarpine by iontophoresis. *Pediatrics* **23**, 545–9.

Kessler, W. R. and Andersen, D. H. (1951). Heat prostration in fibrocystic disease of the pancreas and other conditions. *Pediatrics* **8**, 648–55.

Knowles, M. R., Gatzy, J. T., and Boucher, R. C. (1983*a*). Relative ion permeability of normal and cystic fibrosis nasal epithelium. *Journal of Clinical Investigation* **71**, 1410–17.

Knowles, M. R., Stutts, M. J., Spock, A., Fischer, J., Gatzy, J. T., and Boucher, R. C. (1983*b*). Abnormal ion permeation through cystic fibrosis respiratory epithelium. *Science* **221**, 1067–70.

Knowlton, R. G., et al. (1985). A polymorphic DNA marker linked to cystic fibrosis is located on chromosome 7. *Nature* **318**, 380–2.

Kuzemko, J. A. (1986). Screening, early diagnosis and prenatal diagnosis. *Journal of the Royal Society of Medicine, Suppl. No. 12* **79**, 2–5.

Mearns, M. B. (1969). Discussion on the therapeutic and prophylactic use of mist tents. Proceedings of the 5th International Cystic Fibrosis Conference, p. 153.

Nielsen, O. H. and Schiotz, P. O. (1982). Evaluation of centralized treatment, 1945–1981. *Acta Paediatrica Scandinavia Suppl.* **301**, 107–19.

Phelan, P. and Hey, E. (1984). Cystic fibrosis mortality in England and Wales and in Victoria, Australia 1976–80. *Archives of Disease in Childhood* **59**, 71–83.

Quinton, P. M. and Bijman, J. (1983). Higher bioelectric potentials due to decreased chloride absorption in sweat glands of patients with cystic fibrosis. *New England Journal of Medicine* **308**, 1185–9.

di Sant'Agnesi, P. A., Darling, R. C., Perera, G. A., and Shea, E. (1953). Abnormal electrolyte composition of sweat in cystic fibrosis of the pancreas. *Pediatrics* **12**, 549–63.

Shwachman, H., Kuiczycki, L. L., and Khaw, K. T. (1965). Studies in cystic fibrosis. A report on 65 patients over 17 years of age. *Pediatrics* **36**, 689-9.

Shwachman, H., Kowalski, M., and Khaw, K. T. (1976). *The survival and life style of 70 patients with cystic fibrosis over the age of 25 years.* Proceedings of the VIIth International Cystic Fibrosis Congress, p. 440-2.

Wainwright, B. J. et al. (1985). Localisation of cystic fibrosis locus to chromosome 7cen-q22. *Nature* **318**, 384-5.

Warwick, W. J. (1982). Prognosis for survival with CF: The effects of early diagnosis and CF center care. *Acta Pediatiatrica Scandinavia Suppl.* **301**, 27-31.

Warwick, W. J. and Pogue, R. E. (1969). *Computer studies in cystic fibrosis.* Proceedings of the 5th International Cystic Fibrosis Conference, p. 320-8.

White, R. et al. (1985). A closely linked genetic marker for cystic fibrosis. *Nature* **318**, 382-4.

# 2 Management of cystic fibrosis

J.A. DODGE

## Introduction

Current clinical treatment of cystic fibrosis (CF) is directed towards the prevention or control of the secondary and tertiary manifestations of the disease. At the time of writing, the fundamental physiological defect is still unknown and the prospect of its pharmacological correction is a matter of speculation. Knowledge of the biochemical consequences of the genetic defect would explain why affected individuals are prone to respiratory infection, produce excessive mucus in respiratory and alimentary tract epithelia, lose excessive salt in their sweat, develop pancreatic fibrosis *in utero* and hepatic fibrosis in later life, and are at risk of intestinal obstruction. Some or all of these consequences might be preventable by intervention at one or more points in the biochemical pathway. Until now, treatment has been directed at the consequences of these pathophysiological abnormalities, including, as far as possible, prevention of the lung infection which is the most important tertiary result. Just as basic research has yielded partial answers to enquiries into the nature of CF, with many disappointing false leads, clinical research has resulted in considerable improvement in the life-span of cystic fibrosis patients, despite the fact that from time to time various forms of treatment have been shown to be of no value or even potentially harmful. It should not be forgotten that clinical research must be carried out within strict ethical parameters, the potential benefits of any experimental treatment being carefully weighed against its possible adverse effects. The fact that most cystic fibrosis patients are children who are unable to give legally valid consent for experimental treatments increases the ethical problems associated with research, while at the same time clinicians are aware of the need to start potentially helpful treatment as early as possible, before serious lung damage has occurred. The fact that the mean survival of patients is now measured in decades rather than the few months or years of the early reports is a tribute to the dedication and opportunism of the clinicians who have made a special study of this disease, and ensured that their patients received the benefit of medical advances as they have occurred.

In this chapter I shall describe some of the standard approaches to treatment of the various clinical aspects of cystic fibrosis. Only general principles will be discussed and more detail may be found elsewhere (e.g. Goodchild and Dodge 1985).

## The sweat abnormality

Increased sodium chloride content of the sweat is one of the most consistent biochemical features of cystic fibrosis, and has been the basis of the standard diagnostic test for many years. The salt loss itself is usually of no great importance to the patient, and in temperate climates there is no need for routine supplementation of the diet with extra salt. However, in heat-waves or in the hot, dry summers of southern Europe, children with cystic fibrosis sometimes collapse with heat stroke. This can be prevented by a generous salt intake with meals.

The salt content of the sweat normally rises with age, so that levels which might be considered diagnostic of cystic fibrosis in a young child would be of uncertain significance in an adult. A short course of dexamethasone may clarify the situation, because it significantly lowers the sweat chloride concentration in normal individuals but has little or no effect in those with cystic fibrosis.

## Pancreatic insufficiency

Although pancreatic function is reasonably well preserved in some affected infants, sooner or later the majority develop steatorrhoea as a result of lipase deficiency. There is also malabsorption of protein but carbohydrate absorption is generally satisfactory. Dried extracts of animal pancreas in capsule or tablet form may be taken at meals to compensate for the absence of the patient's own pancreatic enzymes. The various products available differ considerably in their enzyme content and bioavailability. The most satisfactory formulation is one in which individual granules of pancreatin are enteric coated to prevent their inactivation by acid in the stomach. The enteric coating is lost in the duodenum, where the pancreatin is released. Pancreatic enzymes work best in an alkaline medium, but secretion of bicarbonate by the pancreas is nearly always very poor in cystic fibrosis so that the pH may never rise to an optimal level in the small intestine. Sodium bicarbonate can be given with meals, or a histamine-receptor antagonist can be used to suppress gastric-acid secretion. However, these measures are rarely necessary if the dose of pancreatin is adequate, and fat absorption can be improved to nearly normal levels by pancreatin alone.

As life expectancy has increased, so has the incidence of diabetes mellitus. This is presumed to be a complication of increasing pancreatic fibrosis which results in impaired blood supply to the islets of Langerhans and their eventual demise. The diabetes is treated in the standard way, with insulin given according to individual requirements.

## Nutritional problems

Malnutrition was formerly one of the major clinical features of cystic fibrosis in early childhood but modern management has considerably improved growth and development. When adequate replacement pancreatin is given, normal growth and weight gain can be expected. Later, some faltering of growth or loss of weight usually develops. This is generally associated with deteriorating respiratory function and increasing pulmonary infection, but the relationships between various contributory factors are complex. It has been shown that the ratio of weight to height in CF is more closely related to the degree of respiratory disease than to the adequacy of pancreatic function (Kraemer et al. 1978), although the severity of these two major features of CF tends to be similar (Gaskin et al. 1982).

There is a complex interaction of digestive, metabolic, physiological, and adaptive factors which combine to increase the overall calorific requirements to as much as 120–150 per cent of the recommended daily allowance, and even when this level of intake is achieved severe impairment of lung function increases the work of breathing to a point where weight loss or growth failure may be inevitable (Dodge 1988). If body weight or growth are to be maintained in this situation, intensive nutritional rehabilitation using enteral or parenteral methods becomes necessary. Ideally, the child with CF should be growing at a normal velocity along his own genetically determined height and weight centiles, while adults should be maintaining their body weight.

Before efficient pancreatin preparations were available, patients were often advised to take a low-fat diet. The high calorific density of fat meant that they were often depriving themselves of a large proportion of the calories in a normal diet, and this deficiency was not usually adequately compensated for by increases in carbohydrate and protein intake. Moreover, low-fat diets carry a theoretical and probably clinically important risk of producing essential fatty acid deficiency. It has even been proposed that essential fatty acid deficiency can explain some of the pathological features of CF (Carlstedt-Duke et al. 1986). Current nutritional advice to patients includes a recommendation that fat intake should be at least normal, and some centres actually increase the fat intake to boost total calories, while others advise specific supplements of essential fatty acids. Of course, pancreatin supplements must also be increased proportionately.

Fat malabsorption is likely to lead to deficiency of fat-soluble vitamins, such as A, D, E, and K. Case reports of clinical deficiency of all these vitamins have been published, particularly in infancy. Babies with CF detected by neonatal screening methods before clinical symptoms have occurred have been found to have biochemical deficiencies of vitamins A and E already. Standard practice is to advise supplementation with a multi-vitamin product in twice the 'normal' daily dosage, and to give additional supplements of vitamin E. Neurological complications may occur in the long term in vitamin E-deficient individuals.

Deficiencies of trace elements are also sometimes observed. Frank iron-deficiency anaemia is uncommon, although serum iron and ferritin levels are quite often low. It should be remembered that patients with advanced respiratory disease from any cause tend to have a raised haemoglobin, and a level towards the lower end of the normal range may represent true anaemia for that group of patients. Low levels of serum or plasma zinc are not uncommon, while biochemical evidence of selenium deficiency has also been recorded in CF. Long-term selenium deficiency has also been speculatively associated with an increased risk of carcinoma in patients who survive to adult life (Stead *et al.* 1985). However, there is no clinical or other evidence to support the view that cystic fibrosis itself is due to either deficiency or disordered metabolism of selenium, and routine selenium supplementation is not recommended (Dworkin *et al.* 1987).

## Bowel complications

Between 10 and 20 per cent of cases of CF present in the newborn period with meconium ileus. In this condition, the lumen of the distal small intestine is obstructed by tenacious plugs of meconium, and in some cases the distended bowel becomes twisted before birth (volvulus), compromising the blood supply to the bowel or even causing gangrene and perforation. Meconium ileus is an emergency which requires transfer of the baby to a neonatal surgical unit. Operative treatment is often required but in some uncomplicated cases the obstruction can be relieved by an enema of 'gastrografin', a water-soluble iodinated contrast medium. This preparation has high osmolality and has the effect of drawing fluid into the intestinal lumen. Clearly, large amounts of intravenous fluid are required to prevent dehydration, and the procedure requires skill and experience. It should not be undertaken in peripheral centres away from the surgical skills which may be required if the procedure is unsuccessful. Under radiological control, gastrografin is introduced *per rectum* and it passes through the small, unused colon to the point of obstruction. If the procedure is successful, the retained meconium is dislodged and passed within a few hours along with large amounts of fluid and 'gastrografin'. It may be necessary to repeat the procedure.

In those cases where surgical intervention is necessary, i.e. where the diagnosis is in doubt, or there is evidence of volvulus or perforation, the standard operation is known as the Bishop–Koop procedure in which the small bowel is divided, any gangrenous or non-viable gut excised, and the lumen irrigated to remove as much of the inspissated material as possible. The proximal small gut is joined to the distal portion in an end-to-side fashion, and the distal portion brought to the surface as an ileostomy. Continuity is thus retained, and when stools are being passed normally via the colon the ileostomy is closed.

Many older patients complain of abdominal pain, particularly when pancreatic supplementation is inadequate. In some, a mass can be felt in the right lower quadrant of the abdomen, which is sometimes tender. Occasionally, subacute or acute intestinal obstruction occurs and these patients sometimes come to operation when the cause of the problem is not recognized. They are found to have intraluminal obstruction by a thick porridge-like mass in the caecum, ascending colon, and terminal ileum. This condition is sometimes known as 'meconium ileus equivalent', but as there is no meconium or ileus it is more properly referred to as the distal intestinal obstruction syndrome. Like meconium ileus, it can be managed with gastrografin either as an enema or given through a naso-gastric tube. Other agents, such as *N*-acetylcysteine, have also been used successfully, but the most recent and successful treatment is administration by mouth or tube of very large amounts of a balanced intestinal lavage solution ('Golytely').

Invagination of the intestinal tract (intussusception) sometimes occurs in children with CF, and is probably precipitated by inspissated bowel contents blocking the ileo-caecal valve. It may require operative treatment.

Rectal prolapse is an occasional problem of the pre-school child, often associated with bulky stools and malnutrition. Although distressing, it is not serious in itself and the extruded rectal mucosa can be returned through the anus with the child lying down. Prevention is by increasing pancreatic supplements to an effective level.

## Liver disease

Although histological evidence of increased hepatic fibrosis is almost universal in older patients with CF, it is an important clinical problem in less than 10 per cent. With improved survival, the incidence of clinically significant liver disease is expected to rise. Its pathogenesis is uncertain, and prevention therefore impossible. When cirrhosis is established, alcohol and aspirin should be avoided, the former because it may further increase the damage and the latter because it may cause erosion of the gastro-oesophageal mucosa, where varices may be present. Vomiting of blood (haematemesis) may occur spontaneously due to bleeding varices, and is treated conservatively with sedation, intramuscular vitamin K, and fresh blood-transfusion, followed if necessary by intravenous pitressin. Gastric acid secretion should be suppressed by a histamine-receptor antagonist, such as cimetidine or ranitidine. Following an episode of haematemesis, the varices may be injected under direct vision through an endoscope with a sclerosing agent. Several treatments are usually necessary. Rarely, the first haematemesis is so severe that it does not respond to conservative measures and emergency surgical treatment is required, with oesophageal or gastric transection. As patients may have varices for many years before bleeding occurs, there is no indication for routine endoscopy or radiography to determine their presence, even when portal hypertension is suspected because of splenic enlargement.

In a small proportion of patients, liver failure may be the major clinical problem. This is treated along conventional lines, with a high-protein diet and diuretics. Gall-stones are not uncommon, but rarely become symptomatic.

## Respiratory disease

Pathological changes are found throughout the respiratory tract and present by far the most serious problem in most cases.

### Obstruction

Within weeks of birth, mucous glands in the lungs are seen to be distended, and mucus often blocks the small airways, where it stagnates. Infection with bacteria is a common sequel. Later in childhood, and in adult life, many CF patients show increased sensitivity of the bronchi to a variety of challenges—ranging from exercise to inhaled proteins—in other words, they behave like true asthmatics. This component of airways obstruction responds to bronchodilators such as Salbutamol, most effectively given as an aerosol.

Physiotherapy is the cornerstone of the treatment of respiratory disease, and is directed at removing mucus, whether infected or not, from the lungs. Various techniques are employed. They may involve manual percussion of the chest by a physiotherapist, parent, or other helper; deep breathing and forced expiration by the patient himself (forced expiration technique, FET); expiration against positive pressure administered by a mask (PEP mask); chest compression by the patient himself or by an assistant; and postural drainage, in which one or more of these manoeuvres is applied while the patient adopts various body positions in order to drain different parts of the lungs. Most patients need to carry out their physiotherapy two or three times a day, each session taking about 20–30 minutes. Patients of all ages find this irksome and increasingly are looking to alternatives. Regular programmes of exercise, including swimming, running, tennis, and dancing may make the patient cough and bring up retained secretions, but if exercise is to be used as a substitute for physiotherapy, it must be carried out daily.

Nasal obstruction from polyps is common in CF and is occasionally the presenting symptom of the disease. If removed, the polyps nearly always return and, moreover, the anaesthetic required for surgery is itself a hazard, often being followed by a deterioration in lung function (Price 1986). The polyps often become smaller when treated with corticosteroid sprays or drops, and unless both nostrils are completely blocked, which is unusual, surgery is best avoided.

## Infection

Sooner or later, mucus retained in the lungs becomes infected, and infection, once established, is extremely difficult to eradicate. A wide variety of pathogens may be responsible, but those which are encountered most frequently include *Staphylococcus aureus, Haemophilus infuenzae, Pseudomonas aeruginosa, Pseudomonas cepacia*, and certain fungi, such as *Aspergillus fumigatus* and *Candida albicans*. Viruses such as influenza may also affect the lungs, just as in other people, and predispose to secondary infection with bacteria. There is no evidence that the individual with CF is excessively prone to such infections but the consequences are likely to be more serious.

It is obviously desirable to prevent infection from occurring in the first place, and this is one of the strongest arguments for instituting physiotherapy, even in young infants, as soon as the diagnosis is made in order to keep the lungs drained of mucus. Because staphylococcal infection is particularly damaging, and most likely to occur in early life, many physicians treat their young children with continuous narrow-spectrum anti-staphylococcal antibiotics such as flucloxacillin, while others use antibiotics in high dosage at the first sign of a respiratory infection. Immunization against whooping cough and measles is an important part of the care of young children with CF, but immunization against *Pseudomonas* infection has been unsuccessful.

The majority of patients eventually become infected with *Pseudomonas aeruginosa* (Pitt 1986). This organism has relatively low pathogenicity but is almost impossible to eradicate. It gives a characteristic green colour to the sputum, which is often produced copiously. Laboratory cultures often show that several strains of *Pseudomonas* are present at the same time. A highly characteristic feature is the so-called mucoid change, whereby *Pseudomonas* strains isolated from CF patients frequently produce very large amounts of a mucoid exopolysaccharide or alginate when cultured in the laboratory. *Pseudomonas* strains found in CF may be highly sensitive to antibiotics *in vitro* but nevertheless continue to be isolated during and after a full course of appropriate therapy. Treatment of *Pseudomonas* infection is therefore directed towards containment rather than elimination, and there are practical reasons for giving anti-pseudomonal drugs in courses of limited duration.

The antibiotics employed are mostly $\beta$-lactam drugs, such as certain penicillins (carbenicillin, azlocillin) or aminoglycosides (gentamicin, tobramycin, netilmicin), often given in combination. The aminoglycosides have toxic effects on the kidneys and the inner ear, and courses are usually limited to about 14 days. All of these drugs must be given by injection several times a day, and this is most conveniently given through an intravenous line. Recently, another class of drugs, quinolone derivatives such as ciprofloxacin and norfloxacin, have been shown to have powerful anti-pseudomonal activity, and they have the advantage that they can be given by mouth. Unfortunately resistance usually develops within a few weeks, but when treatment is stopped sensitivity usually returns so that further courses can be given.

Some centres have adopted a policy of admitting patients on a regular basis, every few months, for a course of anti-pseudomonal therapy regardless of symptoms. Others treat only acute exacerbations—characterized by weight loss, malaise, deteriorating lung function and X-ray changes, increased cough and sputum, and sometimes pyrexia. The choice of antibiotics is often dictated by *in vitro* laboratory sensitivies, and occasionally limited by allergy to certain drugs. Antibiotics are also widely used by inhalation as aerosols, and have been shown to reduce the frequency of admission for exacerbations of infection when given on a regular basis (Hodson *et al.* 1981).

Secondary infection with fungi is not uncommon, and some patients develop allergic aspergillosis in which severe bronchospasm plays a major role. It usually responds to corticosteriods with or without anti-fungal therapy. Vigorous and frequent physiotherapy is an essential component of any course of treatment.

## Other complications

Streaks of blood in the sputum are not uncommon but occasionally a large blood vessel in the bronchial tree will become eroded and massive haemoptysis occurs. This is a life-threatening emergency: the patient requires blood transfusion and urgent transfer to a large regional centre. Sophisticated radiological techniques or bronchoscopy are used to identify the source of bleeding, and the vessel can be embolized with gelatin foam or a tiny metal coil introduced through an arterial catheter. Rupture of a thin-walled air sac produced by distortion of lung architecture sometimes occurs, particularly in older patients, causing leakage of air into the pleural cavity which builds up to produce tension and compresses the underlying lung (pneumothorax). Some episodes resolve spontaneously but others require insertion of a drainage tube into the pleural cavity. Recurrent pneumothorax may require surgical treatment in which an irritant substance is introduced to produce adhesions between the two layers of pleura.

## Lung transplantation

Heart–lung transplants have been given to a number of young CF adults with advanced lung disease. Early experience was not encouraging, the first British and US recipients dying within 2 months of surgery. Subsequent results have been much better. Although clearly this cannot be a standard approach to treatment of advanced CF, it will probably continue to have a role in well-selected cases. It is interesting—and scientifically important—to note that the characteristic ion transport defect does not develop in the donor lungs, although of course it remains in the nasal mucosa, and in tracheal mucosa above the site of anastomosis (Alton *et al.* 1987).

# Psychological problems

The whole family is involved when the diagnosis of cystic fibrosis is made in a child (Burton 1975). At first, the burden falls particularly on the parents. They must come to terms with the fact that their child has an inherited disorder which they as unwitting carriers have passed on. It is important to explain to them that feelings of guilt are inappropriate. At the same time they have to adjust their expectations for the child to the possibility that his life will be shortened by this disease, for which we have no cure. Nevertheless, a very demanding regimen of treatment will be prescribed, which will interfere with their own lives as well as that of the child. They must also realize that there is a 25 per cent risk that any further child of the marriage will be affected. Sometimes this genetic advice comes when another pregnancy has already been started, while occasionally there is the added blow that an older sib of a newly diagnosed patient, previously thought to have asthma or bronchitis, is another CF victim. The fact that the child has inherited CF from both sides of the family sometimes brings parents together in adversity, but where the parental relationship was already under strain the added burden of a child with CF not uncommonly precipitates further marital problems leading to separation or divorce. Parents go through the familiar sequence of emotions which follow bereavement—in this case loss of the healthy child they had hoped for—and may experience shock, denial, anger, and depression before they can make a realistic adjustment. Anger is directed at themselves and also at medical staff who may have overlooked the diagnosis for some time, particularly when their anxieties may have been dismissed or when lung damage is found to be already present.

Other family members also become involved. Grandparents, particularly when the parents themselves are young, may wish to take over an unreasonable amount of the child's care on the grounds that the parents are unable to cope with this added burden. On the other hand, they may deny the diagnosis or fail to understand the bilateral nature of the inheritance and blame it all on the spouse. Other relatives may wish to know whether they are carriers, and the risk of their future offspring having CF: something which could only be answered empirically until the recent discovery of the gene locus and adjacent polymorphisms.

When the CF child reaches school age, teasing by other children because of persistent cough, poor stature, or offensive flatus may be a problem. If the child has significant lung disease, inability to participate fully in games and other activities may add to the problems. There is a strong tendency for parents to over-protect the affected child, with resultant delay in emotional development and achievement of independence.

Adolescents often experience the same feelings of anger, denial, and depression as their parents had when the diagnosis was made. By that time they are aware of the nature of their disability, and their reduced life expectancy. They may experience difficulty in making close relationships, particularly with the opposite sex. The discovery that they are probably infertile often comes as a shock to young men. Some occupations will be closed to them and unemployment may add its own burden of depression. They may have encountered other young people with cystic fibrosis whose health is worse than their own, and the death of such friends and acquaintances is a further challenge to emotional well being.

Adults who marry may wish for children, but the great majority of males are infertile as a result of congenital blockage of the vas deferens. Fertility in females is also reduced, although many have successfully borne children. The likely effects of pregnancy and the physical demands of raising young children on the mother's health must be kept in mind, as well as the likely duration and extent of her ability to look after them. Finally, there comes the realization that the intervals between treatment are becoming shorter and the courses of treatment themselves less effective. The support of family, friends, and professional staff is then critical, up to and including the stage of terminal care.

It is clear that clinical management of these patients requires an understanding of their problems and those of the family. The help of an experienced social worker is invaluable. Some patients find it easier to discuss their problems with a nurse or physiotherapist than with the doctor. Whatever their clinical condition, patients must be encouraged to express their feelings and helped to develop a positive attitude to treatment.

# Delivery of health care

Because cystic fibrosis is such a complex condition and its treatment so protracted, health care is most effectively given by a team familiar with the many problems which can occur and who have at their disposal a variety of therapeutic interventions. It has been convincingly shown from Denmark and elsewhere that life expectancy is better when treatment is given at such specialized clinics (Nielson and Schiøtz 1982; Warwick 1982). Even when patients live at a long distance from such a centre and their routine care must be provided locally, responsibility can be shared. Annual assessments at the cystic fibrosis clinic may detect early evidence of infection, nutritional deficiencies, or other complications, and give the opportunity for discussion with physiotherapists, dietitians, and social workers with particular experience of CF. Regional clinics should also be able to provide authoritative genetic counselling, heterozygote identification, and prenatal diagnosis.

Neonatal screening programmes are in operation in various parts of the world, based on measurement of pancreatic enzymes in blood spots. Blockage of small ducts in the pancreas by thick secretions occurs before birth and in early neonatal life, resulting in increased absorption of retained pancreatic enzymes such as trypsin and lipase into the circulation. More than 90 per cent of infants with CF have raised levels of serum immunoreactive trypsin (IRT), which can be measured by radio-immunoassay or enzyme-linked assays. It has not yet been proved that such early diagnosis substantially affects morbidity or eventual life expectancy, but the cost of screening can be more than offset by the savings from reduced hospital admissions of affected babies during the first two years of life (Wilcken and Chalmers 1985). Apart from any actuarial benefits, neonatal screening allows parents of affected babies to receive early genetic counselling, and prevents the distress and recriminations which result from diagnostic delay. It is likely that the IRT test, which is not completely sensitive or specific, will be replaced by more effective methods resulting from discovery of the basic genetic abnormality. Of course, screening is of no benefit unless it is followed by close surveillance and an active treatment programme. If and when more fundamental treatment of the CF abnormality becomes available, it should obviously be started as early in life as possible.

# References

Alton, E.W.F.W., Batten, J., Hodson, M., Wallwork, J. Higgenbottom, T., and Geddes, D. (1987). Absence of electrochemical defect of cystic fibrosis in transplanted lung. *Lancet* i, 1137–9.

Burton, L. (1975). *The family life of sick children*. Routledge & Kegan Paul, London.

Carlstedt-Duke, J., Brönnegard, M., and Strandvik, B. (1986). Pathological regulation of arachidonic acid release in cystic fibrosis: the putative basic defect. *Proceedings of the National Academy of Science USA* **83**, 9202–6.

Dodge, J.A. (1988). Nutritional requirements in cystic fibrosis. *Journal of Paediatric Gastroenterology and Nutrition Suppl No 1.*, **7**, 8–11.

Dworkin, B., Newman, L.J., Berezin, S., Rosenthal, W.S., Schwarz, S.M., and Weiss, L. (1987). Low blood selenium levels in patients with cystic fibrosis compared to controls and healthy adults. *Journal of Parenteral and Enteral Nutrition* **11**, 38-41.

Gaskin, K., Gurwitz, D., Durie, P., Corey, M., Levison, H., and Forstner, G. (1982). Improved respiratory prognosis in CF patients with normal fat absorption. *Pediatrics* **100**, 857-62.

Goodchild, M.C. and Dodge, J.A. (1985). *Cystic fibrosis. Manual of diagnosis and management*, (2nd edn). Baillière Tindall, London.

Hodson, M.E., Penketh, A.R.L., and Batten, J.C. (1981). Treatment of chronic *Pseudomonas aeruginosa* infection in patients with cystic fibrosis. *Lancet* **ii**, 1137-9.

Kraemer, R., Rudeberg, A., Hadorn, B., and Rossi, E. (1978). Relative underweight in cystic fibrosis and its prognostic value. *Acta Paediatrica Scandinavica* **67**, 33-7.

Nielson, O.H. and Schiótz, P.O. (1982). Cystic fibrosis in Denmark in the period 1945-1981. Evaluation of centralised treatment. *Acta Paediatrica Scandinavica Suppl.* **301**, 107-19.

Pitt, T.L. (1986). Biology of *Pseudomonas aeruginosa* in relation to pulmonary function in cystic fibrosis. *Journal of the Royal Society of Medicine, Suppl. No. 12*, **79**, 13-18.

Price, J.F. (1986). The need to avoid general anaesthesia in cystic fibrosis. *Journal of the Royal Society of Medicine Supplement No. 12* **79**, 10-12.

Stead, R.J., Redington, A.N., Hinks, L., Clayton, B., Hodson, M. and Batten, J.C. (1985). Selenium deficiency and possible increased risk of carcinoma in adults with cystic fibrosis. *Lancet* **ii**, 862-3.

Warwick, W.J. (1982). Prognosis for survival with cystic fibrosis: the effects of early diagnosis and cystic fibrosis center care. *Acta Paediatrica Scandinavica Suppl.* **301**, 27-31.

Wilcken, B. and Chalmers, C. (1985). Reduced morbidity in patients with cystic fibrosis detected by neonatal screening. *Lancet* **ii**, 1319-21.

# 3 Defects in epithelial ion transport in cystic fibrosis

A.W. CUTHBERT

## Introduction

An increasing number of defects in cellular processes are being found in tissues from subjects with cystic fibrosis. However, the disturbing symptoms experienced by patients result from inappropriate functioning of a few epithelial tissues, particularly those of the respiratory system and those associated with the alimentary canal. It is generally held that deficiencies in the transport of inorganic ions and water across epithelial structures may be responsible for the accumulation of viscid mucus secretions on epithelial surfaces. While definitive evidence for this latter point is not available, clear abnormalities in transepithelial transport processes have been demonstrated in epithelial preparations derived from patients with the disease. These abnormalities are under intense investigation at the present time and will form the major emphasis of this chapter.

Although there have been a number of attempts to produce animal models of CF which might be used to investigate the pathophysiology of the disease, no really satisfactory models have evolved. The most common model is the chronically reserpinized rat (Martinez and Cassity 1985) which demonstrates deficits in the transepithelial handling of chloride in salivary secretion. Although there is overwhelming evidence that chloride handling is abnormal in CF, the exact nature of the lesion is unknown and may not be the same as in reserpine-treated animals.

To date, the most crucial information of how epithelial processes are altered in CF have come from studies on human tissues or cells derived from them. Four epithelial tissues have been critically important; they are those of sweat glands, salivary glands, the pancreas, and the respiratory airways.

## Basic transepithelial transport processes

A basic feature of the active transepithelial transport of ions is that the transported species must cross two barriers in series, the apical and basolateral domains of the epithelial cell. In general, one of these processes is passive while the other requires expenditure of metabolic energy. Epithelial cells are asymmetric, the macromolecular membrane components responsible for transport being distributed in ways to operate a series pump-leak process.

Illustrative of transepithelial transport processes are the mechanisms for sodium and for chloride transport (Fig. 3.1). Sodium is transported when ions cross the apical barrier, moving down an electrochemical gradient into the cell, and diffuse toward the basolateral membrane, where they are extruded from the cell by an ATP-dependent sodium pump. The transepithelial transfer of the sodium cation creates a transepithelial potential with the apical face negative to the basolateral (Fig. 3.1a), creating a favourable gradient for movement of an accompanying anion, usually chloride, moving either through or between the cells.

In different types of epithelia the entry mechanism for sodium varies. In tight epithelia, entry is by specialized channels which are blocked by the pyrazine carboxamide, amiloride. In leaky epithelia, sodium entry is by a variety of coupled processes involving symports, in which sodium enters with chloride (electroneutral transport) or with organic solutes such as amino acids and glucose, or by an antiport, for example a sodium proton-exchanger. In leaky epithelia, the conductance of the intercellular tight junctions is relatively low, so that transepithelial potentials are small. Furthermore, the apical membranes of tight epithelia are impressively impermeable to water, although the property may be modified by hormones, while leaky epithelia are water permeable. Consequently, transepithelial salt transport in leaky epithelia is accompanied by osmotic water movement, so that near iso-osmotic fluid is transported. In tight epithelia, transport of salt and water are dissociated from each other.

In the examples discussed above, cations are transported creating conditions for the transepithelial movement of accompanying anions. In other situations transport is anion-led, cations moving across the tissue by anion drag. Consider a tissue capable of active chloride secretion (Fig. 3.1b). Generally, chloride is moved up its electrochemical gradient into the cell, the energy being derived from that stored in the sodium gradient. A sodium–potassium–chloride triporter, with a stoichiometry of 1,1,2, is used to do this. This triporter can be blocked by loop diuretics, such as frusemide and piretanide. Chloride ions can now pass down their electrochemical gradient through chloride channels in the apical membrane, while sodium ions are expelled from cells by the sodium pump, and potassium ions equilibrate across the basolateral membrane through potassium channels. A transepithelial potential, negative on the apical side, is again created, favouring the movement of an accompanying cation. Strikingly, active sodium absorption and secondarily active chloride secretion are both

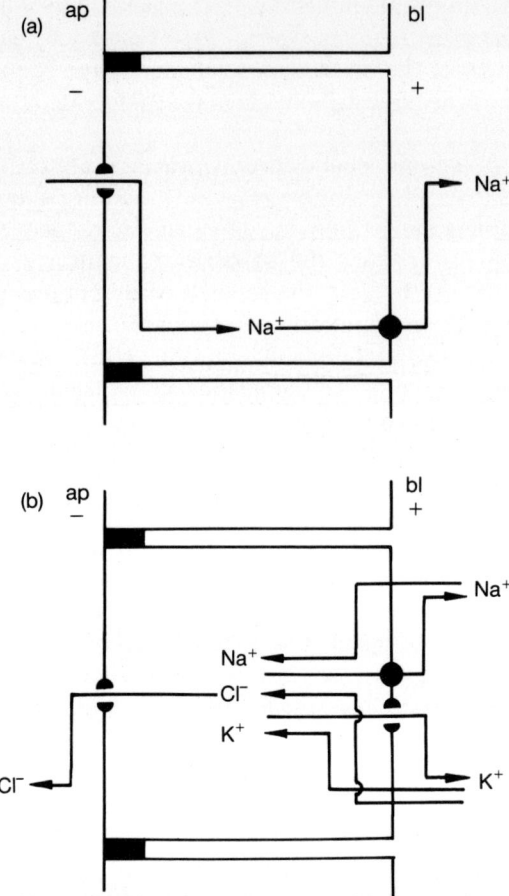

**Fig. 3.1.** Diagrams illustrating transepithelial ion transport processes. Electrogenic sodium absorption is illustrated in (a) and electrogenic chloride secretion is illustrated in (b). Apical membranes (ap) are on the left and basolateral membranes (bl) on the right. Cells are joined at their apical borders by tight junctions. Sodium pumps are shown as filled circles, while various types of ion channels are indicated by breaks in the membranes. Ions pass up or down their electrochemical gradients in moving into or out of the cells as indicated. Note in both transport modes the apical membrane is negative with respect to the basolateral side.

dependent upon a basolateral sodium pump. Chloride secretion in many tissues can be stimulated by agents which increase intracellular cAMP or $Ca^{2+}$. Cyclic AMP increases the chloride permeability of the apical face of the epithelial cells, while $Ca^{2+}$ activates calcium-dependent potassium channels in the basolateral face. The latter serves to increase potassium efflux, to supply the triporter, and to steepen the electrical gradient for chloride exit across the apical face. In many systems, cAMP inhibits electroneutral sodium chloride entry through the apical membrane, while electrogenic chloride secretion is stimulated. Both processes may occur in the same cells or separately, for example intestinal crypts are secretory while the villus epithelium is absorptive.

In general, tight epithelia are located downstream of leaky ones, for example the sweat gland absorptive duct compared to the secretory coil, the colon compared to the intestine, so that fine control of salt and water homeostasis, often under hormonal control, can be achieved in regions where separate handling of salt and water movement is possible.

## Transport abnormalities in cystic fibrosis

### Sweat glands

Useful reviews of the ion transporting characteristics of normal sweat gland epithelia are by Sato (1977), Bijman (1987), and Quinton (1987). Essentially, a near-isotonic sodium chloride solution is formed by the secretory coil of the sweat gland, while the sensible perspiration emanating from the duct is hypotonic, due to salt reabsorption in the duct. The concentration of sodium chloride in sweat depends on flow rate. The processes responsible for the formation of the primary secretion and the removal of salt are those described earlier, namely electrogenic chloride secretion in the coil and electrogenic sodium absorption in the ductal regions. In CF there are defects in both the secretory and absorptive processes of sweat formation, but the consequences are far more pronounced in the latter, giving rise to sweat with a high salt concentration. This phenomenon is unknown except in CF, so that sweat composition has become a crucial diagnositc test for the presence of the disease. Sweat composition in patients with CF compared to controls at comparable sweating rates is given in Table 3.1. When reabsorptive ducts are perfused *in vitro* with 150 mM NaCl, control ducts have a transepithelial potential of around 7.0 mV (lumen negative) while in CF ducts the value is around 77 mV. However, normal ducts also show the same potential when perfused with isotonic sodium sulphate, the sulphate ion being impermeable (Quinton 1983; Bijman and Quinton 1984). Calculation of the permeability ratio, $P(Na)/P(Cl)$ gave a value of 0.26 in controls, compared to 2.3 for CF ducts. It is therefore to Quinton that we owe the first indication that the

**Table 3.1.** Sweating rate, composition, and calculated reabsorption for single sweat glands in CF and controls (Adapted from Quinton and Bijman 1983)

|  | Sweating rate nl/min | Concentration (mM) Na | Cl | Reabsorption rate (pM/min/gland) Na | Cl |
|---|---|---|---|---|---|
| Cf | 2.12 | 93 | 97 | 101 | 48 |
| Controls | 2.26 | 23 | 20 | 252 | 208 |

aberrant handling of chloride is a fundamental defect in CF. The increased transepithelial potential in the CF reabsorptive duct is readily understood by reference to a simple electrical equivalent of the process outlined by Fig. 3.1a (Fig. 3.2). The circuit represents a resistive barrier, $Ra$, in the active pathway and a shunt resistance, $Rs$, in the passive pathway.

The potential, $V$, across the circuit, representing the transepithelial potential, is given by $ERs/(Ra+Rs)$. As $Rs$ becomes very large $V$ and approaches $E$. In the sweat duct, chloride is the counter ion following the actively transported sodium and if chloride conductance is low, as in CF, (i.e. $Rs$ is large), the potential will be greater than in normal glands. Data with the chloride-channel blocking agent, 3',5-dichloro-diphenylamine-2-carboxylic acid, suggests that chloride channels are in the apical membranes of sweat duct cells (Bijman *et al.* 1987). Recently, a number of groups have cultured

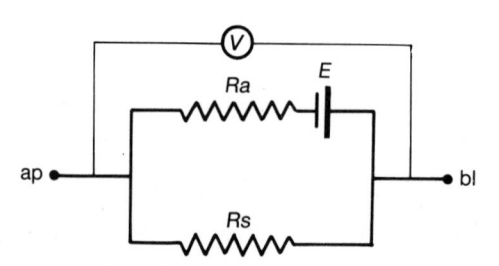

**Fig. 3.2.** Equivalent circuit for active sodium absorption. Resistance, $Ra$, controls the current in the active pathway while $Rs$ controls the passive pathway. The open circuit potential is given by $ERs/Ra+Rs$. If $Rs$ is very large the transepithelial potential, $V$, approaches $E$. An epithelium under open circuit conditions transfers sodium chloride from the apical to the basolateral side. However, if the resistance encountered by the counter ion ($Cl^-$) is high, the rate of transfer will be small. Alternatively, if $Rs$ is small $V$ is much less than $E$ but sodium chloride absorption is increased. Under short-circuit conditions (i.e. $V$ controlled at zero by a voltage clamp) then the short-circuit current ($SCC$) is given by $E/Ra$, that is there is no current flow through $Rs$ and $SCC$ is equivalent to the net sodium flux.

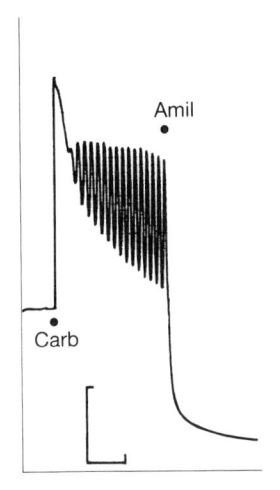

**Fig. 3.3.** Short-circuit current across a cultured epitherlial sheet (area 0.2 cm²) derived from human sweat-gland cells. The preparation has properties of the ductal epithelium and responds to cholinoceptor agonists, such as carbachol. The increase in current is due to an increase in electrogenic sodium absorption. Tissues from both normal and CF patients can be used for comparative studies of transporting activity and sensitivity to drugs (D. Brayden, unpublished). Carb, indicates 10 μM carbachol, applied to the basolateral side of the tissue; Amil, indicates 10 μM amiloride, applied to the apical side of the tissue. Calibrations are 2 μA and 5 min.

sweat gland epithelia on permeable supports so that transepithelial transport processes may be more readily studied. Pedersen and Larsen (1986), using cultures of absorptive ducts, studied the movement of chloride ions when the epithelia were polarized, by an external current, at −50 mV (lumen negative). Chloride currents were found to be greater in normals compared to CF, further β-adrenoceptor stimulation, with isoprenaline, was ineffective in increasing chloride conductance only in CF-derived tissues. Cultures of secretory coil or from whole sweat glands also develop ductal characteristics (Brayden *et al.* 1988). Figure 3.3 shows the response of a whole-gland culture to a cholinoceptor agonist, carbachol. This agent, like acetylcholine, causes an increase in active sodium reabsorption in sweat ducts. The change in phenotypic behaviour in culture indicates the pleuripotential properties of cells from sweat-gland coil.

The secretory coil of human sweat glands can respond to stimuli which affect both β-adrenoceptors and muscarinic cholinoceptors. From a physiological point of view, the latter are most important, the maximal secretory rate per gland being four times that obtained by β-receptor activation (Quinton 1987). The secretory coils of CF glands are abnormal in failing to respond to isoprenaline, while responses to acetylcholine are normal (Sato and Sato 1984). In a recent study (Behm *et al* 1987) it was shown that CF heterozygotes also show a deficient sweating response to β-receptor agonists compared to controls. This is an important finding as it means that heterozygote tissues may be useful in investigation of the cellular lesion in CF. From the foregoing, primary sweat formation is relatively unimpaired in CF, so that sweating rates are similar. While both coil and duct show abnormal responses to stimuli which increases cAMP, cAMP generation is normal in CF secretory coils, indicating a defect downstream of this, resulting in failure to increase the chloride conductance. Cholinoceptor agents are thought to act by a phosphatidylinositol hydrolysis mechanism linked to muscarinic receptors, leading to an increase in $Ca_i$ (intracellular ionized Ca). It is not known if the same cells or cell types can respond both to acetylcholine and catecholamines. Sweat glands in CF are deficient in nerves showing immunoreactivity of vasoactive-intestinal polypeptide (Heinz-Erian *et al* 1985). It is unclear as yet whether this is a primary or secondary effect.

## Airway epithelia

A variety of human airway epithelia has been used in CF research, i.e. tracheal epithelium, that covering nasal polyps removed in polypectomies, and nasal turbinate epithelium removed for plastic or reconstructive considerations. These tissues have been investigated both *in vivo* and *in vitro*. In the latter condition they have been used intact, as isolated cell suspensions, or as primary epithelial monolayers grown on either permeable or impermeable substrates. The essential findings are similar for the different tissues and different situations, so that an overall picture of the functional defects in CF airway epithelia has emerged.

Airway epithelia both absorb and secrete ions. Active sodium transport provides the driving force for fluid absorption from airways; this is particularly important at term in the neonate, where the process may be under hormonal control, and also in the adult situation. In the latter, a reduction in fluid volume is necessary as ciliary action drives fluid into the upper respiratory tree with its ever decreasing surface area.

Secondary active chloride secretion is demonstrable in airway epithelia in response to a variety of neurotransmitters and autacoids, such as acetylcholine, catecholamines, VIP (vasoactive intestinal polypeptide), 5Ht (5-hydroxytryptamine), histamine, kinins, etc. The extent of the fluid layer covering the surface of the airways will depend on the balance between absorptive and secretory processes, excessive absorption or lack of secretion producing a drying effect.

The transepithelial potential across airway epithelia in CF patients is greater than in controls. *In vivo* nasal and tracheal potentials show significantly greater reductions when superfused with amiloride in CF compared to controls. Oppositely, the potential changes are smaller in CF subjects, when the surface is bathed in gluconate-rather than chloride-containing solutions, compared to controls. These results can be interpreted to mean that sodium transport is enhanced in CF while chloride conductance is reduced (Knowles *et al.* 1981, 1983*a*). Note that, using the equivalent circuit given in Fig. 3.2, a decrease in *Ra* and an increase in *Rs* mimics the changes referred to above. These observations have been confirmed using direct measurements of ion flux in excised nasal epithelium *in vitro* (Knowles *et al.* 1983*b*). Further nasal epithelium from normal or atopic individuals, *in vitro*, exhibits electrogenic chloride secretion in response to the β-receptor agonist, isoprenaline, but without changing the extent of electrogenic sodium absorption. In contrast, β-adrenoceptor stimulation of CF nasal epithelium caused no chloride secretion but increased sodium absorption (Yankaskas *et al.* 1985). Thus, like the sweat-gland epithelium, there appears to be a low chloride conductance with an associated lesion such that signals, operating through the cAMP system, fail to increase chloride permeability. Additionally, cAMP is able to increase electrogenic sodium absorption in CF tissues. The latter feature is unusual in mammalian tissues, except perhaps fetal lung (Olver *et al.* 1986) but is common in epithelia in other chordates (e.g. amphibia). Ways of inducing cAMP-sensitive sodium absorption in mammalian epithelia have been explored (Cuthbert and Spayne 1983).

The findings with intact nasal epithelium *in vitro* have been duplicated with primary cultures of tracheal and nasal epithelium grown on permeable supports. Again, chloride secretory responses were small or absent, even though tissue generation of cAMP was normal in CF derived tissues. Increasing $Ca_i$, however, did produce chloride secretion in these monolayers, indicating that the apparatus for chloride secretion was intact, although it could not be triggered by cAMP (Widdicombe 1986). By using glass microelectrodes the effects of isoprenaline on the apical membrane potential and fractional resistance of cultured monolayers of CF and normal tracheal epithelium were measured (Widdicombe *et al.* 1985). The fractional resistance is given by $Ra/(Ra + Rb)$ where *Ra* and *Rb* are respectively the resistance of the apical and basolateral membranes. In normal tissue, isoprenaline reduced both the fractional resistance and membrane potential, while no effect was seen in CF tissues. This locates the lesion to a place which results in a failure of the apical chloride channel to respond to raised intracellular cAMP. In CF airway epithelia, the apical membrane potential showed a greater hyperpolarization and a greater change in transepithelial resistance on application of amiloride compared to controls, indicating increased apical sodium permeability in CF tissues (Cotton *et al.* 1987). Thus, increased sodium absorption and reduced chloride secretion, likely to lead to a drying effect on airway surfaces, result from abnormal functioning of the apical membranes.

The most significant advances in relation to the physiological lesion in CF has come from patch clamp studies (Fig. 3.4). A fire-polished glass microelectrode is lowered onto the surface of a cell where it forms a tight electrical seal (gigaseal). As the area under the electrode is very small (a few $\mu m^2$) only a few channels are included. Currents through individual channels can be measured using sophisticated amplification techniques. It is possible to study the membrane patch in a cell-attached situation or after the patch has been torn from the cell. Characteristically, channels are either open or closed and, at a given membrane voltage, single-channel currents are constant in magnitude. Channel open times and closed times show variations, and statistical analysis of these allow kinetic schemes for channel mechanisms to be deduced.

It is important to realize that patch clamping in the cell-attached and

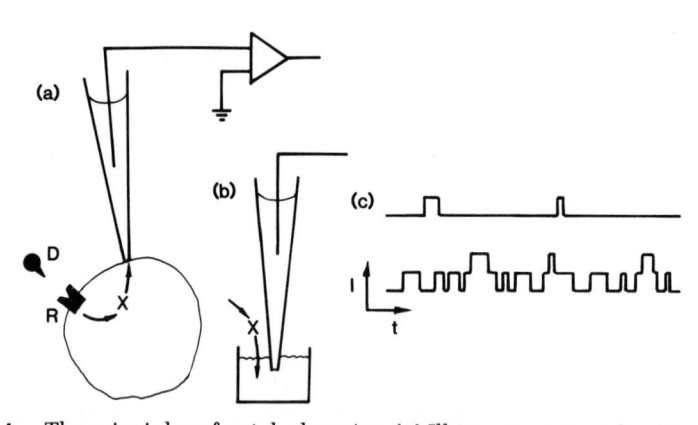

**Fig. 3.4.** The principles of patch clamping. (a) Illustrates principle of the whole-cell recording technique. A glass microelectrode is used to form a gigaseal on the surface of a cell. Records are made by high-resolution recording techniques from the patch under the microelectrode, which includes only a few ion channels. If a drug, D, acting via a receptor, R, alters the probability of channel opening then a diffusible messenger, X, generated within the cell must diffuse to the inner surface of the patch. (b) Alternatively, an isolated patch, pulled off the cell, can be dipped into solutions containing agents which affect the probability of channel opening. (c) Idealized diagram of channel opening and closing. The patch is held at an appropriate potential and single channel currents (openings shown upwards) are shown against time, t. Note single channel currents (and hence conductance at a fixed potential) are constant, while opening times are variable. The upper record represents spontaneous channel opening while the lower record illustrates the effect of an agent which increases the probability of channel opening. Presumably the patch contains only two channels, which occasionally are open at the same time, i.e. when the current amplitude doubles.

isolated-patch configurations give different types of information. Drugs applied to the whole cell cannot reach recognition sites in the patch under the microelectrode tip. If agents increase channel activity in the whole-cell configuration then messengers must diffuse to the channels in the patch. In the isolated patch the solutions bathing both sides can be controlled.

There have been a number of patch clamping studies of the apical membranes of primary cultures of human airway epithelial cells. Chloride channels were identified from the selectivity for chloride over cations and impermeant anions. Chloride channels showed rectification, conductance increasing with outward currents. At zero transepithelial potential two types of channels with conductances of around 25 pS and 50 pS were observed. Chloride channel blockers (e.g. anthracene-9-carboxylate) apparently reduced the single-channel currents, but it is likely that this represents high-frequency blocking and unblocking at a rate greater than the frequency response of the amplifiers.

Isoprenaline, cAMP, or forskolin (an activator of adenylate cyclase) applied to tissues with recording in the cell-attached mode increased the probability of channel opening. In CF monolayers of none of these agents was able to cause activation of chloride channel opening. A23187, a calcium ionophore, however, could activate channels in both normal and CF cultures. More remarkably, isolated patches, ripped from cells, showed identical chloride channel activity, whether or not the patches were derived from CF tissue (Frizzell *et al.* 1986, Welsh 1986; Welsh and Liedtke 1986).

It appears, therefore, that CF cells have normal chloride channels which fail to be triggered by cAMP, although elevating $Ca_i$ does cause chloride channel opening. The appearance of channel activity in isolated patches might be due to the loss of a diffusable inhibitor when the internal membrane face is exposed. Results similar to these are now accruing from patch clamp studies on sweat-gland secretory cells (Schoumacher *et al.* 1987*a*). Finally, exposure of isolated patches from CF tissues to the catalytic subunit of protein kinase A failed to activate channels, indicating that the lesion is downstream of this step (Schoumacher *et al.* 1987*b*). Preliminary investigations suggest that placental trophoblast membranes also have reduced $Cl^-$ permeability compared to normal controls (Davis *et al.* 1985).

## Salivary glands and the pancreas

Recently a method has been described for the culture of interlobular duct cells from the human fetal pancreas (Harris and Coleman 1987). These can be passaged and will undoubtedly be useful for biophysical and biochemical studies. It will be important to establish if the patters of response in this tissue show the same types of defect as do sweat ducts and airway cells. Fragments of human salivary (submandibular) glands from CF subjects show a much depressed response to $\beta$-adrenoceptor stimulation compared to controls.

Activation of the receptors with isoprenaline caused release of both amylase and mucin (McPherson *et al.* 1985, 1986).

## Other systems

### Intestinal epithelia

A number of cell lines derived from colonic adenocarcinomas have been increasingly used for transport studies. Examples are T84 (Dharmasathaphorn *et al.* 1984), Caco-2 (Grasset *et al.* 1984), and HCA-7 (Cuthbert *et al.* 1985). All these lines show electrogenic chloride secretion in response to a variety of secretagogues. There is the occasional report of adenocarcinomas in CF patients (Roberts *et al* 1986) but as yet no cell lines from such sources have been reported. Nevertheless, three cell lines, all derived from the same adenocarcinoma, may yield useful insights in relation to CF. The lines, HCA-7, Colony 1, and Colony 3 respond to a variety of signals which either elevate cAMP or $Ca_i$ (Cuthbert *et al.* 1987), the foremost of these reacting to both types of signal. Colony 1 monolayers, however, show small responses to elevated $Ca_i$ and exaggerated responses to cAMP, while Colony 3 monolayers have the reversed sensitivity (Fig. 3.5). Thus, Colony 3 cells show characteristics of the CF pheontype. Further, it was shown that the failure to respond to signals (e.g. VIP) acting through cAMP was not due to lack of adenylate cyclase, cAMP accumulation, or cAMP-sensitive protein kinase. As these cells are immortalized the problems usually associated with obtaining CF tissues are circumvented.

## Other cell types

Because of the difficulties of obtaining CF epithelia, attempts have been made to use more readily obtainable cells to study the functional lesion. Some details of some of these are given below.

### Red cells and lymphocytes

As $Ca_i$ plays a crucial role in excitation–secretion coupling, many investigators felt that this parameter may be altered in CF. Both in red cells (Muallem *et al.* 1985) and lymphocytes (Grinstein *et al.* 1984) cytosolic calcium concentrations have been found to be normal. However, in red cells, at least, there was a reduction in the number of active calcium pumps (measured as $(Ca^{2+} + Mg^{2+})$ – ATPase activity) but this was associated with a lower rate of passive entry for calcium. Deficiency in the functioning of the Na–K–2Cl co-transporter of CF red cells has also been reported (Brayden *et al.*, 1986). Lymphocytes and granulocytes from CF patients showed a reduced cAMP response to stimulation with isoprenaline. Interestingly,

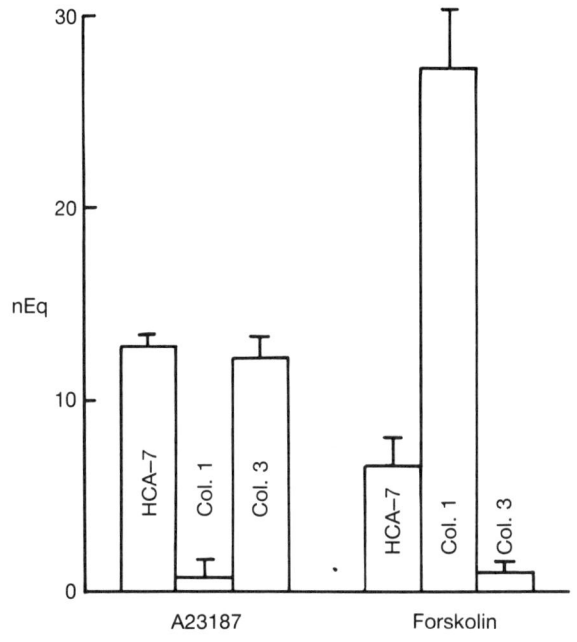

**Fig. 3.5.** Chloride secretory responses (nEq in 8 min) in cultured monolayers (0.2 cm$^2$) of human colonic epithelial cells in response to A23187 (1 μM) or forskolin (10 μM). The three cell lines, HCA-7, Colony 1, and Colony 3 were all derived from the same human colonic adenocarcinoma. The secretory responses result from an increase in Ca$_i$ (with A23187) or cAMP (with forskolin). Each column shows the mean value and standard error from six experiments. Note that Colony 3 cells fail to respond to forskolin, even though this agent causes a significant increase in intracellular cAMP.

heterozygotes showed intermediate responses between CF and normal cells (Davis 1986).

## Fibroblasts

In cultured skin fibroblasts intracellular chloride is contained in two compartments, which can be demonstrated by efflux studies. Apparently the chloride content in both of these compartments is reduced in CF (Mattes et al. 1987). A number of calmodulin-binding proteins can be detected in both normal and CF skin fibroblasts. Binding of [125]I-calmodulin to the 46.5 kD protein was reduced in CF fibroblasts, indicating either reduced availability or affinity (Tallant and Wallace 1987).

## Other hypotheses

Much evidence is accumulating, both for transporting epithelia and other systems, that there are complex interactions between different second-messenger systems. Details of these interactions are beyond the scope of this review. Various hypotheses have been put forward to explain how the basic defect in CF operates to affect physiological function, often involving interactions of second-messenger systems and sometimes invoking dependence on various signalling mechanisms, such as autonomic effectors and the eicosanoids. These hypotheses are useful in formulating new experiments but, as yet, they have not led to new insights. Examples are hypotheses based on altered functions of calmodulin (Rupp 1986; McPherson and Dormer 1987) or defective regulation of prostaglandin formation or function (Anderson 1984; Carlstedt-Duke *et al.* 1986).

## New approaches

One way in which the study of altered physiology in CF tissues would be greatly facilitated would be the availability of immortalized cell lines would preserve the CF phenotype. A number of groups are attempting to produce such lines for experimental work.

An alternative way to study epithelial ion channels and their regulation is to induce the channels in other cells which are experimentally amenable. The *Xenopus* oocyte is a convenient cell into which mRNA from normal and CF tissues can be injected. There is a preliminary report that $Cl^-$ uptake into oocytes injected with CF mRNA was reduced compared to controls injected with mRNA from normal tissues (Grzesiuk and Carroll 1987).

## Unknowns

Most of the references quoted in this review are from the past three years, which might give the impression that considerable advances have been made in understanding the physiological defect. While there is cause for optimism, there are many unknowns. For example, it is not yet known if vectorial transport of macromolecules or the composition of these is altered in CF. While some might hold that the viscid mucin secretion characteristic of CF is a consequence of abnormal ion transport, others maintain that the secretion is abnormal. Similarly, it is not yet known if the defects in bicarbonate secretion in the pancreas have the same basis as deficiencies in chloride secretion elsewhere, or indeed, if bicarbonate ions can pass through chloride channels. The failure, as yet, to detect abnormalities in chloride transport in the kidney is surprising, while abnormalities in acid–base transport have been reported in affected epithelia. Finally, there is no definitive evidence to show whether the susceptibility to infection of the airways is related to an abnormal ion composition, mucin accumulation, or both.

## Opportunities for therapeutic strategies

Making assumptions about the role of abnormal ion transporting activities in CF epithelia, it is possible to formulate hypotheses for a treatment. For example, failure in the regulation of epithelial chloride channels is almost certainly due to a defective intracellular process. Rather than correct this process, it is possible to consider developing agents which will regulate the chloride channel from outside the cell. Thus far only chloride channel blockers are available, but these might form lead compounds for chloride channel agonists.

In the airways, deficiencies in chloride secretion are exacerbated by excessive sodium absorption. The amiloride series of drugs are specific blockers of epithelial sodium channels and topical amiloride is currently undergoing clinical trial in CF patients (Waltner *et al.* 1987). Coupling of amiloride to large polymers (e.g. dextrans) by the permissive part of the molecule (Cuthbert 1976) might confine the drug to the pulmonary system and prevent systemic effects.

## Note added in proof

A recent report shows that intestinal epithelia in CF respond neither to cAMP or Ca mediated secretagogues, unlike airway epithelia (Berschneider *et al.*, 1988).

## References

Anderson, C. M. (1984). Hypothesis revisited. Cystic Fibrosis: A disturbance of water and electrolyte movement in exocrine secretory tissue associated with altered prostaglandin (PGE$_2$) metabolism? *Journal of Pediatric Gastroenterology and Nutrition* **3**, 15–22.

Behm, J. K., Hagiwara, G., Lewiston, N. J., Quinton, P. M., and Wine, J. J. (1987). Hyposecretion of β-adrenergically induced sweating in cystic fibrosis heterozygotes. *Pediatric Research* **22**, 271–6.

Berschneider, H. M., *et al.* (1988). Altered intestinal chlorider transport in cystic fibrosis. *FASEB Journal* **2**, 2625–9.

Bijman, J. (1987) Transport processes in the eccrine sweat gland. *Kidney International* **32**, (Suppl. 21), S109–S112.

Bijman, J. and Quinton, P. M. (1984). Influence of abnormal Cl$^-$ impermeability on sweating in cystic fibrosis. *American Journal of Physiology* **247**, C3–C9.

Bijman, J., Englert, H. C., Lang, H. J., Greger, R., and Fromter, E. (1987). Characterisation of human sweat duct chloride conductance by chloride channel blockers. *Pflugers Archiv. European Journal of Physiology* **408**, 511–14.

Brayden, D., Martin, U., Ryan, M.P., Brady, H., and Fitzgerald, M.X. (1986). Reduced loop diuretic-sensitive $^{86}$Rb influx in red blood cells of cystic fibrosis patients. *British Journal of Pharmacology* **87**, 50P.

Brayden, D., Cuthbert, A.W., and Lee, C.M. (1988). Human eccrine sweat gland epithelial cultures express ductal characteristics. *Journal of Physiology* **405**, 657-75.

Carlstedt-Duke, J., Bronnegard, M., and Strandvik, B. (1986). Pathological regulation of arachidonic acid release in cystic fibrosis. The putative basic defect. *Proceedings of the National Academy of Sciences USA* **83**, 9202-6.

Cotton, C.U., Stutts, M.J., Knowles, M.R., Gatzy, J.T., and Boucher, R.C. (1987). Abnormal apical cellmembrane in cystic fibrosis respiratory epithelium. An *in vitro* electrophysiological analysis. *Journal of Clinical Investigation* **79**, 80-5.

Cuthbert, A.W. (1976). Importance of guanidinium groups for blocking sodium channels in epithelia. *Molecular Pharmacology* **12**, 945-57.

Cuthbert, A.W. and Spayne, J.A. (1983). Conversion of sodium channels to a form sensitive to cyclic AMP by component(s) from red cells. *British Journal of Pharmacology* **79**, 783-97.

Cuthbert, A.W., Kirkland, S.C., and MacVinish, L.J. (1985). Kinin effects on ion transport in monolayers of HCA-7 cells, a line from a human colonic adenocarcinoma. *British Journal of Pharmacology* **86**, 3-5.

Cuthbert, A.W., Egleme, C., Greenwood, H., Hickman, M.E., Kirkland, S.C. and MacVinish, L.J. (1987). Calcium- and cyclic AMP-dependent chloride secretion in human colonic epithelia. *British Journal of Pharmacology* **91**, 503-15.

Davis, B., Sharman, D.B., and Boyd, C.A.R. (1985). Chloride transport in cystic fibrosis placenta. *Lancet* **i**, 392-3.

Davis, P.B. (1986). Physiological implications of the autonomic aberrations in cystic fibrosis. *Hormone and metabolic Research* **18**, 217-20.

Dharmasathaphorn, K., McRoberts, J.A., Mandel, K.G., Tisdale, L.D., and Masin, H. (1984). A human colonic tumour cell line that maintains vectorial electrolyte transport. *American Journal of Physiology* **246**, G204-G208.

Frizzell, R.A., Rechkemmer, G., and Shoemaker, R.L. (1986). Altered regulation of airway epithelial cell chloride channels in cystic fibrosis. *Science* **233**, 558-60.

Grasset, E., Pinto, M., Dessaulx, E., Zweibaum, A., and Desjeux, J.F. (1984). Epithelial properties of human colonic carcinoma cell line Caco-2: electrical properties. *American Journal of Physiology* **2477**, C260-C267.

Grinstein, S., Elder, B., Clarke, C.A., and Buckwald, M. (1984). Is cytoplasmic $Ca^{2+}$ in lymphocytes elevated in cystic fibrosis? *Biochimica et Biophysica Acta* **769**, 270-4.

Grzesiuk, E. and Carroll, D. (1987). Transplantation to frog oocytes of the chloride permeability defect associated with cystic fibrosis. *Pediatric Pulmonology* Suppl. 1, Abstract 20.

Harris, A. and Coleman, L. (1987). Establishment of a tissue culture system for epithelial cells derived from the human pancreas: a model for the study of cystic fibrosis. *Journal of Cell Science* **87**, 695-703.

Heinz-Erian, P., Dey, R.D., Flux, M., and Said, S.I. (1985). Deficient vasoactive intestinal peptide innervation in the sweat glands of cystic fibrosis patients. *Science* **229**, 1407-8.

Knowles, M., Gatzy, J., and Boucher, R. (1981). Increased bioelectric potential

difference across respiratory epithelia in cystic fibrosis. *New England Journal of Medicine* **305**, 1489-95.
Knowles, M., Gatzy, J., and Boucher, R. (1983*a*). Relative ion permeability of normal and cystic fibrosis nasal epithelium. *Journal of Clinical Investigation* **71**, 1410-17.
Knowles, M.R., Stutts, M.J., Spock, A., Fischer, N., Gatzy, J.N., and Boucher, R.C. (1983*b*). Abnormal ion permeation through cystic fibrosis respiratory epithelium. *Science* **221**, 1067-70.
McPherson, M.A. and Dormer, R.L. (1987). The molecular and biochemical basis of cystic fibrosis. *Bioscience Reports* **7**, 167-85.
McPherson, M.A., Dormer, R.L., Dodge, J.A., and Goodchild, M.C. (1985). Adrenergic responses of submandibular tissues from control subjects and cystic fibrosis patients. *Clinica Chimica Acta* **148**, 229-37.
McPherson, M.A., Dormer, R.L., Bradbury, N.A., Dodge, J.A., and Goodchild, M.C. (1986). Defective β-adrenergic secretory responses in submandibular acinar cells from cystic fibrosis patients. *Lancet* **i**, 1007-8.
Martinez, J.R. and Cassity, N. (1985). The chronically reserpinized rat as a model for cystic fibrosis: Abnormal chloride transport as the basis for reduced salivary fluid secretion. *Pediatric Research* **19**, 711-16.
Mattes, P.M., Maloney, P.C., and Littlefield, J.W. (1987). Altered chloride metabolism in cultured cystic fibrosis skin fibroblasts. *Proceedings of the National Academy of Sciences* **84**, 3009-13.
Muallem, S., Miner, C., and Seymour, C.A. (1985). The nature of the $Ca^{2+}$-pump defect in the red blood cells of patients with cystic fibrosis. *Biochimica et Biophysica Acta* **819**, 143-7.
Olver, R.E., Rasmden, C.A., Strang, L.B., and Walters, D.V. (1986). The role of amiloride-blockable sodium transport in adrenaline-induced lung liquid adsorption in the fetal lamb. *Journal of Physiology* **376**, 321-40.
Pedersen, P.S. and Larsen, H.V. (1986). Chloride flux studies in normal and cystic fibrosis sweat duct cell cultures. *IRCS Medical Science* **14**, 1159-60.
Quinton, P.M. (1983). Chloride impermeability in cystic fibrosis. *Nature* **301**, 421-2.
Quinton, P.M. (1987). Physiology of sweat secretion. *Kidney International* **32**, (Suppl. 21), S102-S108.
Quinton, P.M. and Bijman, J. (1983). Higher bioelectric potentials due to decreased chloride absorption in the sweat glands of patients with cystic fibrosis. *New England Journal of Medicine* **308**, 1185-9.
Roberts, J.A., Tullett, W.M., Thomas, J. St. J., Galloway, D., and Stack, B.H.R. (1986). Bowel adenocarcinoma in a patient with cystic fibrosis. *Scottish Medical Journal* **31**, 109.
Rupp, G.M. (1986). The pathogenesis of cystic fibrosis. A proposal for calmodulin as the basic biochemical defect. *Medical Hypotheses* **20**, 245-53.
Sato, K. (1977) The physiology, pharmacology and biochemistry of the eccrine sweat gland. *Reviews of Physiology, Biochemistry and Pharmacology* **79**, 52-131.
Sato, K. and Sato, F. (1984). Defective beta adrenergic response of cystic fibrosis sweat glands *in vivo* and *in vitro*. *Journal of Clinical Investigation* **73**, 1763-71.
Schoumacher, R.A., Shoemaker, R.L., and Frizzell, R.A. (1987*a*). Abnormal regulation of apical membrane chloride channels in sweat gland secretary cells in cystic fibrosis. *Federation Proceedings* **46**, 1272.

Schoumacher, R. A., Shoemaker, R. L., Halm, D. R., and Frizzell, R. A. (1987b). Activation of chloride channels in airway cells by the catalytic subunit of A-kinase and membrane depolarisation. *Pediatric Pulmonology*, Suppl. 1, Abstract 33.

Tallant, E. A. and Wallace, R. W. (1987). Altered binding of $^{125}$I-labelled calmodulin to a 46.5 kilodalton protein in skin fibroblasts cultured from patients with cystic fibrosis. *Journal of Clinical Investigation* **79**, 643-8.

Waltner, W. E., Boucher, R. C., Gatzy, J. T., and Knowles, M. R. (1987). Pharmacotherapy of airway disease in cystic fibrosis. *Trends in Pharmacological Science* **8**, 316-19.

Welsh, M. J. (1986). The apical-membrane chloride channel in human tracheal epithelium. *Science* **232**, 1648-50.

Welsh, M. J. and Liedtke, C. M. (1986). Chloride and potassium channels in cystic fibrosis airway epithelia. *Nature* **322**, 467-70.

Widdicombe, J. H. (1986). Cystic fibrosis and β-adrenergic response of airway epithelial cell cultures. *American Journal of Physiology* **251**, R818-R822.

Widdicombe, J. H., Welsh, M. J., and Finkbeiner, W. E. (1985). Cystic fibrosis decreases the apical membrane chloride permeability of monolayers cultured from cells of the tracheal epithelium. *Proceedings of the National Academy of Sciences USA* **82**, 6167-71.

Yankaskas, J. R., Cotton, C. U., Knowles, M. R., Gatzy, J. T., and Boucher, R. C. (1985). Culture of human nasal epithelial cells on collagen matrix supports. A comparison of bioelectric properties of normal and cystic fibrosis epithelia. *American Review of Respiratory Diseases* **132**, 1281-7.

# 4 Molecular genetics

VERONICA VAN HEYNINGEN and
DAVID J. PORTEOUS

## The molecular approach to genetic disease

It is a basic tenet of molecular biology that mutation at the DNA level underlies the phenotypic changes seen at the level of the whole organism in genetic disease. Identification and isolation of the gene at the disease locus provides a reliable clinical diagnostic tool and, ideally, a precise understanding of the metabolic consequences of the mutation. This may open up possibilities for therapeutic intervention.

Cystic fibrosis (CF) is a genetic disease which exhibits simple Mendelian inheritance in affected families (McKusick, 1986) and therefore a molecular biological approach can be used to attempt defining the mutant gene. Despite great effort and ingenuity, biochemical and physiological analyses have failed to reveal the metabolic basis of the disease (Talamo *et al.* 1983; Chapter 3). Many of the observed deviations from normal must be secondary to the basic defect. The ultimate test for identifying the disease gene is perfect cosegregation of molecular genotype with the disease phenotype in affected families.

The advent of recombinant DNA technology (the cloning, restriction mapping, and DNA sequencing of segments of the human genome) permit us to study DNA structure down to the single nucleotide level. Restriction enzymes (which recognize DNA sequence with strict accuracy) reveal a great deal of individual variation at the DNA level, far more frequent and often more clearcut than those observed at the protein level. Genetic analysis is totally dependent on our ability to find and follow individual differences ('markers') within families. This task is made simple by looking at the DNA level with techniques which are rapidly becoming routine lab practice. Many, or even most, cloned sequences, whether or not they encode a protein, will reveal 'restriction fragment length polymorphisms' (RFLPs) in the population (Weatherall 1985; Wright 1986). In this way maternal and paternal copies of markers can be followed within families. Application of this new technology to genetic disease is an extremely powerful tool for defining the mutant gene.

Here we describe the progress that has been made over the past few years in the search for the *CF* gene. Points of principle will occasionally be illustrated by reference to data on other genetic diseases. It will become obvious that the molecular genetic approach is here to stay, but that the 'old' biochemical and cell-biological techniques must continue as a necessary complement to the new technology. We still need to seek confirmation from basic biochemical analyses in reaching a complete definition of genetic disease states.

The two major approaches to identifying the *CF* gene are:

1. Classical genetics: the testing of candidate genes, suggested by biochemical or physiological observations of the disease process, for co-segregation, and therefore identity, with the *CF* gene.

2. Reverse genetics: the use of random markers assigned to each autosome to seek genetic linkage with the *CF* gene. Once this has been achieved, a variety of somatic cell and molecular genetic techniques come into play in moving from linked markers to the gene.

The accurate chromosomal localization of the *CF* gene has been accomplished by establishing linkage to random, functionally unrelated, markers. The second stage of moving from linked marker to the gene is now in progress. There are a number of different approaches being applied to this difficult step of traversing what, in genetic terms, is a very small distance, but in DNA terms is still immense. Recognizing when we have arrived may be the hardest part of all. It is at this stage that all the accumulated biochemical and physiological evidence pertinent to the nature of the basic defect must be re-examined to ensure that the identity and function of the *CF* gene fits in with the observed phenotype.

Whatever the approach, we rely absolutely on the availability of DNA from informative families.

## Family studies

### The genetics of cystic fibrosis

The recurrence risk of CF is 1 in 4 in families with a previous affected child. This autosomal recessive pattern of inheritance is one of the most complex to analyse because heterozygotes, who only carry one copy of the mutant gene, are clinically indistinguishable from normal individuals who carry two copies of the wild-type gene. The parents are obligate heterozygotes, with an average 2 out of 3 of the clinically normal offspring being carriers (Fig. 4.1).

Unless the heterozygotes can be distinguished from normals by some biochemical or physiological means, inheritance of the *CF* gene can only be followed from parents to homozygous affected child. This means that only families with more than one affected child can be informative for the co-

Molecular genetics 43

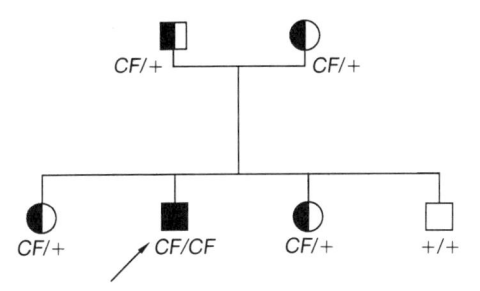

```
         CF/+ ☐─┬─◐ CF/+
                │
      ┌─────────┼─────────┬─────────┐
      ◐        ■         ◐         ☐
     CF/+    ↗ CF/CF    CF/+      +/+
```

Fig. 4.1. The theoretically expected segregation pattern in a family with an affected CF child (arrowed).

segregation of the CF gene with other markers. The greater the number of affected sibs available for analysis, the higher the informativeness of the family.

## Segregation analysis to map a disease locus

If a large number of polymorphic markers, positioned at regular intervals along the chromosomes, is available then segregation analysis carried out in informative affected families should allow us to define the chromosomal location of the mutant disease gene (Solomon and Bodmer 1979; Botstein et al. 1980). Polymorphic differences of any measurable type can be utilized. Thus protein analysis at structural (e.g. electrophoretic mobility) or functional (e.g. variation in enzyme activity) level can be carried out (Harris 1980). At the DNA level, variations in position, or presence and absence, of specific restriction sites in the genomic DNA will be revealed in Southern blots (Weatherall 1985) as fragments of different molecular weight (RFLPs) hybridizing with the marker probe. A clear advantage of DNA analysis is that DNA from any available cell type can be used, while only a proportion of protein gene products are expressed in any one cell type. A third approach, which on rare occasions yields results in linkage studies, is cytogenetic analysis. Some disease loci can be associated regularly or sporadically, with clearly segregating chromosomal abnormalities such as deletions or translocation breakpoints (e.g. Cri-du-chat syndrome, sporadic aniridia, or Duchenne muscular dystrophy in females). No such cytogenetic association has been found in CF.

It should be pointed out that for clearcut linkage between disease locus and marker(s) to be established, it is important to be sure that there is no genetic heterogeneity observed for the disease, i.e. that the mutation is present at the same locus in all cases. Statistical analysis of disease occurrence patterns at the population level can reveal heterogeneity or confirm homogeneity. Variability at the clinical level may be an indication of genetic diversity, as demonstrated for haemophilia (Graham et al. 1983), xeroderma pigmentosum (Hashem et al. 1980), or the mucopolysaccharidoses (Neufeld and Fratantoni 1970; McKusick 1986). Conversely, it seems that Duchenne and Becker muscular dystrophies, which are considered clinically quite distinct entities, probably map to the same large gene locus (Forrest et al. 1987). Cystic fibrosis does exhibit clinical variability: for example, not all patients suffer from pancreatic insufficiency (Sing et al. 1982; Talamo et al. 1983). Accurate and detailed diagnosis is essential. However, an observation which suggests that CF is caused by non-complementing mutation(s) in a single gene, is that the frequency of cousin–cousin marriages among the parents of CF patients in Italy is not significantly different from that expected for a single locus recessive disorder (Romeo et al. 1985).

## Classical genetics and assessment of candidate genes

There is a long, amply documented (Talamo et al. 1983) history of the search for biochemical and physiological abnormalities in CF. Because so many reports failed the test of repeatability, any which showed some degree of consistency were explored as candidates in family studies. The repeated observation of the presence in CF patients of serum factors or proteins which inhibit ciliary motion in a variety of assays (Bowman et al. 1969; Conover et al. 1973) made these factors early candidates for the *CF* gene. The presence of these factors in the clinically normal heterozygote as well as in affected individuals strengthened the possibility that whatever gene codes for the ciliary dyskinesis factor is the *CF* gene. Suggestions emerged that a proteolytic cleavage fragment of complement component C3 might be the ciliary dyskinesis factor (Conover et al. 1974). As soon as a genomic fragment clone for the *C3* gene became available this hypothesis could be tested and rejected on the basis that polymorphic alleles of *C3* do not co-segregate with CF in two informative families (Davies et al. 1983; and Fig. 4.2). A tenuous hint (Mayo et al. 1980) that the gene for ciliary dyskinesis factor resides on chromosome 4 triggered considerable efforts to test this hypothesis by family segregation analysis, and resulted in chromosome 4 being one of the first to be excluded as the site of the *CF* gene (Scambler et al. 1985).

One of the observations which has been confirmed in several laboratories (Nevin et al. 1981; Brock et al. 1982; Grataroli et al. 1984) has been the demonstration, on isoelectric focusing of serum from CF patients and from obligate heterozygotes, of a pI 8.4 doublet band which is not seen in normal individuals (Wilson et al. 1975). The nature of the protein and its possible relationship to the dyskinesia factors remained an enigma for years. Eventually Manson and Brock (1980) produced an antiserum to protein excised from the isoelectric focusing gel. This made possible antigen quantitation by rocket immunoelectrophoresis which revealed a high level of cystic fibrosis

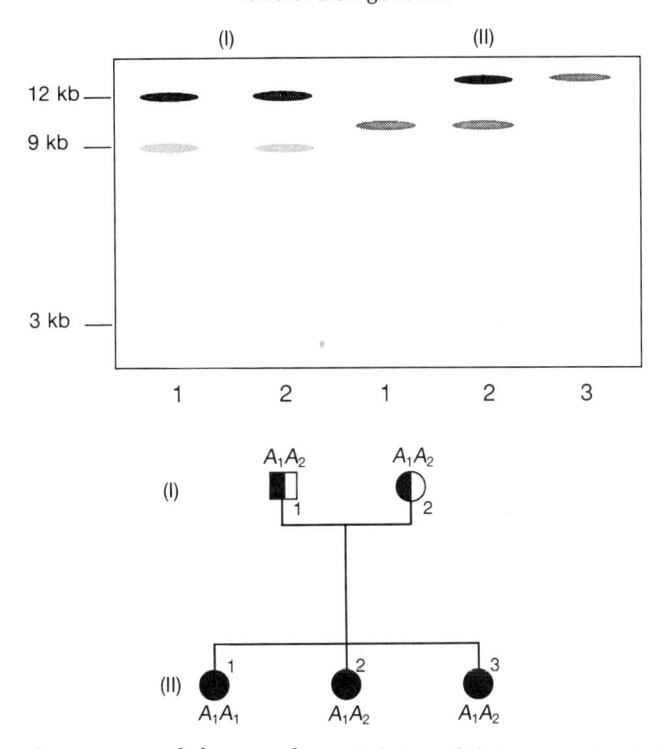

**Fig. 4.2.** Assessment of the complement *C3* candidate gene for tight linkage (identity) with the *CF* gene in a family with three affected children. The upper panel is a diagrammatic interpretation of the DNA blot analysis in family members I1, I2, II1, II2, II3. The lower panel is a pedigree diagram with the interpretation of the data showing a complete lack of concordant segregation between the *CF* gene and alleles of the *C3* gene in this family. (Data from Davies *et al.* 1983, with permission.)

antigen (CFAG) in CF patients, an intermediate level in heterozygotes, and no detectable antigen in normals. This pattern of expression suggested that CFAG might be the product of the defective *CF* gene or that it acts within the CF pathway as an intermediate or effector which accumulates in a gene dose-dependent manner. We therefore set out to map and identify the gene coding for CFAG. With the aid of somatic cell hybrids capable of expressing this granulocyte differentiated cell product, we succeeded in assigning the *CFAG* gene to chromosome 1 (van Heyningen *et al.* 1985*a*). At this stage chromosome 1 was still a candidate for the location of the *CF* gene (see 'Human gene mapping 8' 1985), but soon after this, the primary defect was unequivocally assigned to chromosome 7 (see below). However, the possibility of a functional relationship between the disease gene product and

CFAG remained. We therefore continued efforts to identify the CFAG protein by conventional molecular biological approaches (Dorin et al. 1987). Monoclonal antibodies raised against CFAG have allowed us to immuno-purify the protein, which was then subjected to $N$-terminal amino-acid sequencing. From this sequence the possible nucleotide sequences that could code for a small part of the protein were deduced and synthesized as a series of oligonucleotide probes. These probes were used to screen a cDNA library which we had constructed from messenger RNA derived from myeloid cells where we knew CFAG was actively synthesized. One clone was verified, from the partial amino-acid sequence for CFAG, as carrying the coding sequence for *CFAG*. Comparison of the complete amino-acid sequence (deduced from the experimentally determined nucleotide sequence) with all sequences of proteins with known functions in the database, revealed homology to a family of calcium-binding proteins. The possible relationship of such a protein with the basic defect in CF is under investigation. It is interesting to note that one member of the homologous gene family has been shown to be the regulatory subunit of a hetero-tetrameric protein which is the phosphorylation target for the activated epidermal growth factor receptor and for other similar cellular signalling systems. Such signal transduction pathways probably participate in the control of ion-channel opening which has been shown to be abnormal in affected epithelia in CF (Welsh and Liedtke 1986; Frizzel et al. 1986). Components of such pathways are plausible candidates for the defective *CF* gene product.

The promise of a reliable heterozygote detection assay which had been held out by the early data on CFAG quantitation (Manson and Brock 1980; Brock et al. 1982) has not been realized when further, more exhaustive, analyses were carried out with the aid of the monoclonal antibodies to CFAG (Hayward et al. 1987), because there is too much overlap between CFAG levels in the three genotypes. Heterozygote detection remains an important aim in the prevention of CF, but may only become feasible once the *CF* gene and its product are identified.

As a result of physiological studies on ion transport (Chapter 3) a number of candidates for the *CF* gene have been suggested; for some of these, DNA clones are available. Once the chromosomal localization of the *CF* gene had been accomplished (*v.i.*), candidate genes could be tested for co-localization. For example, the mapping of the gene encoding the non-erythroid homologue of the Band 3 protein (which in red cells mediates the exchange of chloride and bicarbonate ions across the cell membrane) to chromosome 7 was tantalizing, but sub-localization to band 7q35–36, some distance from the *CF* gene (Palumbo et al. 1986), excluded this from being the *CF* gene. Similarly, calmodulin, which is a calcium-binding protein implicated in the regulation of many calcium-dependent cellular functions, has been excluded as the product of the *CF* gene by several criteria (Scambler et al. 1987*a*).

# Reverse genetics

## Segregation analysis to link the CF gene with random markers

The haploid human genome is $\sim 3 \times 10^9$ nucleotide base pairs (bp) long. This is equivalent to a total genetic map length of 3000 cM (Renwick 1969). Setting out to find the location of a disease gene by linkage to a known marker is a daunting task. Nevertheless, with the advent of RFLP analysis, several groups felt that it was feasible to attempt to define the position of the *CF* gene locus by family linkage studies, using both DNA and protein polymorphic markers. As discussed earlier, only homozygous affected individuals (a minimum of two per family) and their obligate carrier parents can be informative in such an analysis, although the statistical significance of results can be improved by inclusion of data on unaffected sibs and grandparents (White *et al*. 1985*a*). The process of finding firm linkage between a disease locus and any other defined marker depends on the possibility of distinguishing repeated co-segregation of an allele at the marker locus with the disease. The likelihood of discerning such a pattern in the limited number of available families is greatly increased if the linked marker is multi-allelic, i.e. one with a high polymorphism information content (PIC value) (Botstein *et al*. 1980). Work is now in progress to clone and map a series of high PIC value probes to cover the whole genome with evenly spaced (about 10 cM apart) markers for more efficient linkage analysis (Solomon and Bodmer 1979; Botstein *et al*. 1980). However, it was with much painstaking labour that by August 1985 ('Human gene mapping 8' 1985) about 40 per cent of the genome was said to be excluded from linkage with the *CF* locus. The reliability of such a claim was, of course, not known. One major problem in assessing this is that most of the markers used had been assigned to their chromosomal position by means of physical mapping techniques (e.g. using deletion and translocation breakpoints or by *in situ* hybridization to metaphase chromosomes). Even now, the relationship of physical to genetic map distance is not clear, but it seems likely that it varies with chromosomal location: there are recombinational hot spots and cold spots so that 1 cM is not equivalent to the same number of base pairs everywhere along the chromosome (van Heyningen and Porteous 1986). Positive data are much more reliable. The first significant linkage of the *CF* locus with a marker was reported at this same workshop (Eiberg *et al*. 1985*a, b*). Unexpectedly, the association, at a recombination fraction of 0.1 (map distance 10 cM) with a LOD score of 2.7, was with the polymorphic serum enzyme paraoxonase (*PON*) rather than with a cloned DNA fragment.

## From first linkage to chromosomal site of the CF gene

The next problem to be overcome was that *PON* itself had not been assigned to a chromosome. It was still necessary to define the location of the *CF* locus by mapping *PON* or by finding other assigned or assignable markers which could be shown to be linked both to *CF* and to *PON*. Chromosomal localization of a gene encoding an enzyme activity is a complex procedure requiring segregation analysis with already assigned markers either in family studies or using somatic cell hybrids capable of expressing the function. It is therefore not surprising that the next polymorphic marker reported to be linked to *CF* was a cloned single-copy genomic DNA sequence *D7S15*, defined by the probe DOCRI-917 (Tsui *et al.* 1985). *D7S15* was found to be 15 cM from the *CF* locus and 5 cM from *PON*. Fast on the heels of the assignment of this probe to chromosome 7 by somatic cell hybrid analysis (Knowlton *et al.* 1985) came the announcement of two much closer markers. The cellular oncogene *MET* was shown by White *et al.* (1986b) to be tightly linked (0–5 cM, maximum LOD = 8.65) to the *CF* locus, segregating here in a different set of families from Utah. Simultaneously, Wainwright *et al.* (1985) reported equally close linkage in the London series of CF families, with an anonymous chromosome 7 marker *D7S8* defined by probe pJ3.11. Sub-chromosomal localization of these linked probes placed the *CF* locus between bands q22 and q32 on the long arm of chromosome 7. Other previously assigned chromosome 7 genes for the T-cell receptor beta subunit (*TCRB*) and for collagen alpha I (*COL1A2*) could also be shown to be *CF*-linked at greater genetic distances than *MET* or *D7S8* (see Bowcock *et al.* 1986). The combined physical and genetic map of chromosome 7 at this stage is shown in Fig. 4.3a.

## Immediate usefulness of linked markers

The availability of two RFLP markers within a few centimorgans of the disease gene immediately raised the possibility of following the mutant *CF* gene within families with a previous affected child (from whom DNA is available). Prenatal diagnosis at the DNA level was quickly offered (Farrall *et al.* 1986a). The detection of *CF* gene carriers within families also became possible (Farrall *et al.* 1986b). Details of the procedures used are described in Chapter 5. Obviously, with a two-allele system at each linked locus only some families would be informative (Porteous and van Heyningen 1986). Partly to generate further markers for family studies, and partly to define in more detail the chromosomal region around the *CF* gene, a number of chromosome 7 assigned polymorphic probes were tested for linkage with the disease. Some were found to be sufficiently closely linked to be informative in tracking the *CF* gene in families (Estivill *et al.* 1986, Scambler *et al.* 1986a). The evolving chromosome 7 map at this stage is shown in Fig. 4.3b.

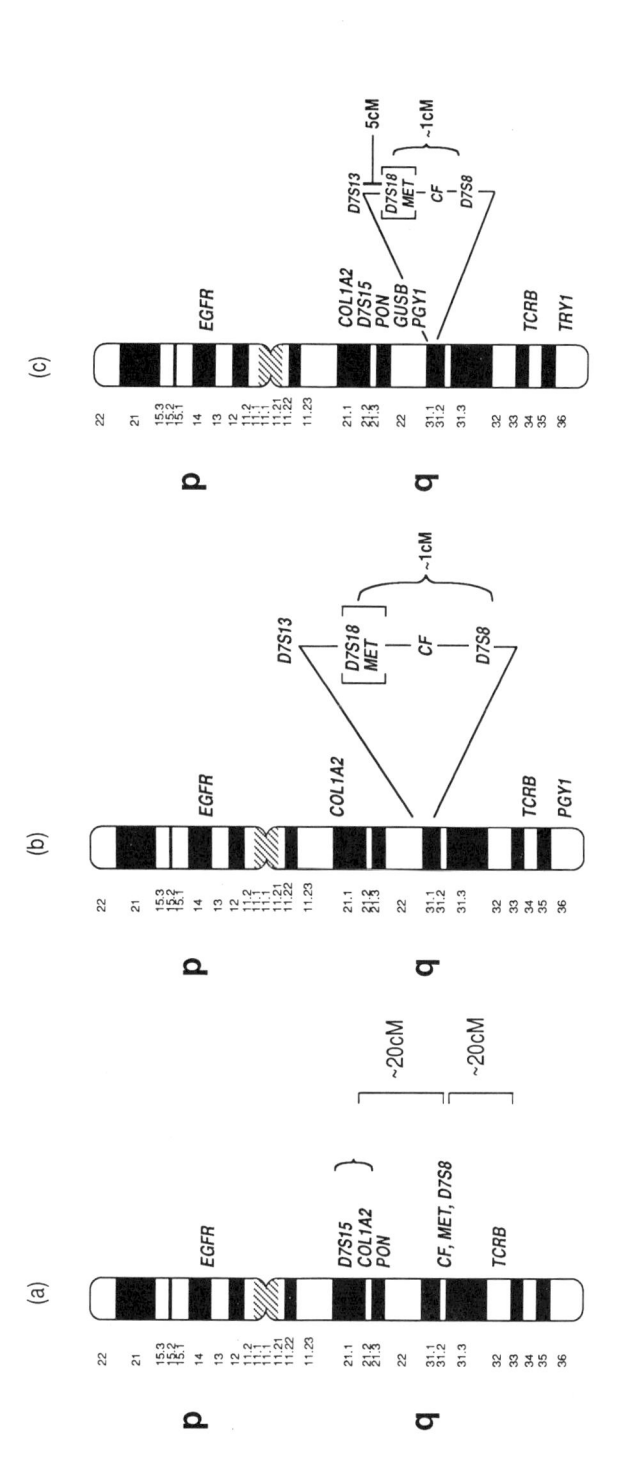

**Fig. 4.3.** The evolution of the chromosome 7 map in relation to the localization of the *CF* gene (see text). (a) The earliest DNA marker assignments. (b) New markers inserted and genetic distances refined near the *CF* locus. (c) Order of markers deduced from a combination of somatic cell hybird analysis and family segregation analysis.

The observation that two different chromosome 7 markers co-segregate very closely with the *CF* gene in families collected over geographically wide areas (see Beaudet *et al.* 1986) supports the suggestion (Romeo *et al.* 1985) that there is considerable, or even complete, genetic homogeneity for mutation at a single *CF* locus. Knowing that there is virtually no heterogeneity means that a statistically much more significant genetic linkage map can be derived by combining results on families around the world (Beaudet *et al.* 1986; Schmidtke *et al.* 1987). Gene order with respect to the disease locus and closely linked markers can only be deduced from a large body of family data.

The linked markers can also be used to establish a physical linkage map for the long arm of chromosome 7. One way of achieving this is by marker analysis of deletion and translocation breakpoints available for the appropriate chromosome region. No disease-associated chromosomal anomalies have been reported for CF. Therefore, physical mapping is only possible for the linked markers relative to each other but not to the *CF* locus, and using random available breakpoints. Although it is possible to carry out dosage analysis of deletion cell DNA by comparing the number of copies of the test marker to a second marker known to be present at diploid copy number (van Heyningen *et al.* 1985*b*; Wainwright *et al.* 1987), this technique is difficult if many probes need to be tested. More reliable and clean data can be obtained from the more laborious technique of somatic cell hybrid analysis (van Heyningen *et al.* 1985*b*). Translocation as well as deletion chromosomes with informative breakpoints can be selectively retained in rodent–human cell hybrids in the absence of the normal homologue, and DNA from such cells is analysed for the simple presence or absence of the human-specific restriction fragments detected by each marker. Such an analysis has been carried out for the *CF* locus-linked markers by Zengerling *et al.* (1987), whose results are incorporated in the chromosome 7 marker map in Fig. 4.3c.

Once a disease locus has been so closely defined, the way is open to generate other, more informative, more closely linked probes and to move from linked marker to the gene itself.

## From linked markers to the gene

To set out on this journey, it is necessary to have some idea of the physical distance (in DNA terms) to be covered and of the direction from each marker to the disease locus. Although the genetic distance of the two closest markers to the *CF* gene, *MET* and *D7S8*, is better defined as more CF families are analysed for segregation at these loci (Beaudet *et al.* 1986; Schmidtke *et al.* 1987), the distance in terms of DNA is not known. The reason for this is our ignorance of the relationship between genetic and physical distance. As discussed above, on average, 1 cM is equivalent to $10^6$ bp. However, from cytogenetic observations of chiasma frequency (Hulten 1974) in meiosis

Molecular genetics 51

when recombination takes place, and from linkage studies with physically accurately localized probes, it seems highly likely that recombination occurs unevenly along the length of chromosomes. The tips of chromosomes (van Heyningen and Porteous 1986) and perhaps some specific interstitial sites (Steinmetz et al. 1986) appear to be recombinational hot spots. This could mean that in the CF region (at the middle of the chromosome arm) distances are larger, or indeed smaller, than average.

The exact gene order of the linked markers to the CF gene and to each other is very difficult to establish unequivocally (Beaudet et al. 1986; Schmidtke et al. 1987). This requires allele analysis in informative recombinant families which are by definition a very small percentage of the total. For example: recombination may be expected in 0.7 per cent of meioses for the CF-MET interval, and to help define gene order for CF, MET, and D7S8, the individual in whom cross-over has taken place must be a phase-known heterozygote for D7S8 alleles (Fig. 4.4). With a fair number of informative families analysed, it is now accepted that D7S8 and MET are flanking markers to the CF locus. The evolving techniques of 'reverse genetics' are being used to confirm gene order, and to tackle the problem of physical distance as well as the cloning of the gene itself.

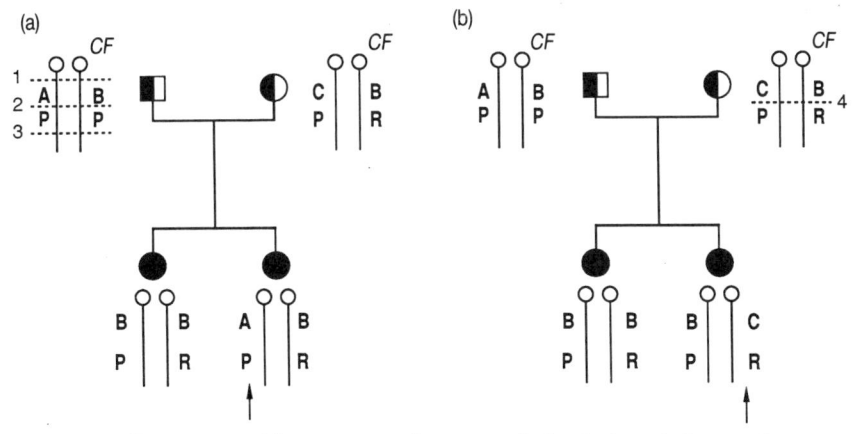

Fig. 4.4. Illustration of how gene order can only be deduced if recombination takes place in an individual doubly informative for at least two heterozygous linked markers. (a) In this pedigree the two affected offspring have different genotypes such that recombination must have taken place in the father. The same recombinant paternal chromosome AP (marked with arrow) can be obtained with cross-over positions (marked ---) at 1, 2, or 3, depending on the site of the CF locus along the chromosome. The recombinant genotype gives no information about the position of the disease locus relative to the markers. (b) If the same parents had two affected offspring with the different genotypes shown, then recombination must have taken place in the doubly heterozygous mother. In this case the cross-over position must lie between the two markers and the CF allele is at a locus centromere-distal to the recombination site at 4.

## Reverse genetics and the new technologies

As soon as the precise location of the *CF* gene on human chromosome 7 was established, several alternative but complementary somatic cell and molecular genetic approaches for 'homing in' on the primary defect were suggested (Porteous and van Heyningen 1986). All of these 'reverse genetic' approaches (Orkin 1986) for moving from linked markers towards the disease gene have since been tested, each with a measure of success. Obviously, each strategy has been tailored to tackle the CF problem, but all are adaptable to the solution of comparable problems for other genetic diseases. A brief outline of the various methodologies is therefore warranted.

### Pulsed field gel electrophoresis (PFGE)

Conventional agarose gel electrophoresis (where application of a constant, unidirectional voltage permits resolution to DNA molecules only up to $\sim 50$ kbp in size) is not amenable to the construction of long-range maps which link adjacent but non-contiguous DNA segments. This impasse has recently been overcome in spectacular fashion with the advent of a new type of gel electrophoresis which relies upon discontinuous electric fields (commonly referred to as 'pulsed fields') to mobilize and resolve very large DNA fragments (Schwartz and Cantor 1984). Several variants on the original theme have been described (see Anand 1986). Each method has its particular attributes and peculiar idiosyncracies. Considerable advances and refinements have been made in the few years since the first description of the methodology, largely as a result of the enthusiasm of those working in the field of molecular medicine. Originally developed to study the DNA structure of intact yeast chromosomes (which in *S. cerevisiae* range in size from $\sim 250$ kbp to $\sim 2.5$ Mbp), the technique is being applied more and more to the molecular analysis of the human genome. For the moment, it is not possible to resolve even the smallest intact human chromosome, but megabase-sized, sub-chromosomal fragments can be analysed. Pulsed field gel electrophoresis can therefore be used to construct long-range restriction maps spanning genetically linked markers (see Barlow and Lehrach 1987). In this way it may be possible to define a large restriction fragment which carries markers closely flanking a disease locus and hence the site of the disease gene itself.

New ways for handling such long lengths of DNA, by embedding cells in agarose blocks to minimize shearing forces, allow chromosomal lengths of DNA to be prepared. Restriction endonucleases specific for sequences which occur only rarely in the human genome (Table 4.1) can then be used to digest this DNA *in situ*. The discrete sub-chromosomal lengths of DNA so generated can now be resolved by PFGE. The 'rare cutter' enzyme sites most often contain one or more CpG dinucleotides, a pairing which is under-

**Table 4.1.** Characteristics of 'rare cutter', enzymes (adapted from Lindsay and Bird (1987); see text for further details)

| Enzyme | Site | Sites per genome ($\times 10^{-4}$) Bulk DNA | Sites per genome ($\times 10^{-4}$) Islands | Percentage of sites in islands | Sites per island |
|---|---|---|---|---|---|
| NotI | GCGGCCGC | 0.05 | 0.36 | 89 | 0.12 |
| EagI | CGGCCG | | | | |
| SacII | CCGCGG | 1.2 | 3.5 | 74 | 1.2 |
| BssHII | GCGCGC | | | | |
| SmaI | CCCGGG | | | | |
| NaeI | GCCGGC | 4.8 | 3.5 | 42 | 1.2 |
| NarI (NunI) | GGCGCC | | | | |
| MluI | ACGCGT | 2.7 | 1.0 | 27 | 0.34 |
| PvuI | CGATCG | | | | |

represented in mammalian genomes, probably due largely to the susceptibility of the cytosines to methylation and subsequent mutation to thymidine (Bird 1986). It happens that these 'rare cutter' sites are frequently found to be associated with coding sequences, as a consequence of the 'islands' of undermethylation characteristic of the 5' ends of housekeeping genes (Bird 1986; Lindsay and Bird 1987). Consequently, PFGE analysis with 'rare cutter' enzymes can generate a gene-to-gene restriction map, with genetically tightly linked but non-contiguous DNA segments co-hybridizing to the same large DNA fragment. Not surprisingly, application of this technology and interpretation of the results is not without its drawbacks (Barlow and Lehrach 1987). For instance, it has proved difficult to map *D7S8* and *MET* to the same restriction fragment.

The details of the PFGE map around the *CF* region are still being worked out. Estimates for the *D7S8-MET* distance are being refined (Poustka *et al.* 1988; Drumm *et al* 1988). Resolving and accurately sizing these large molecules will improve steadily with experimentation and experience. A more serious problem is generation of the DNA markers necessary to link up adjacent 'rare cutter' sites on the chromosome. Recognition of this problem has led directly to the development of two new strategies for genomic library construction.

## 'Jumping' and 'Linking' libraries

Conventional lambda and cosmid cloning vectors can accept individual fragments of human DNA with sizes of up to ~20 kbp and ~50 kbp, respectively. It is at least theoretically possible to make extensive, overlapping genomic libraries in such vectors and, starting with the flanking markers *D7S8* and *MET*, search for independent but partially overlapping clones and thus initiate a 'walk' towards the *CF* gene. In practice, the longest successful 'walks' have fallen far short of even the genetically tiny distance separating *D7S8* and *MET* from *CF*. There are several reasons for this. The average size of each step tends to fall far short of the vector cloning capacity, so that progress is more at a 'shuffle' than a 'walk'. There is also the problem of unclonable sequences and of segments of repeated DNA sequences blocking further progress. Nor is there any directionality to the 'walk'; the chances of moving away from or towards the *CF* gene are equal.

'Jumping' and 'linking' libraries seek to overcome the limitations of conventional libraries for long-range mapping exercises and are specifically designed to interact with PFGE analysis (Poustka and Lehrach 1986). Both have been applied to the CF problem (Collins *et al.* 1987; Michiels *et al.* 1987).

In conventional library construction, linear DNA molecules of a size appropriate for direct insertion into the cloning vector are prepared by restriction with a suitable endonuclease. To construct a 'jumping' library (Fig. 4.5) digestion with a 'rare cutter' enzyme is used to generate a set of very large linear DNA fragments. Next, the linear molecules are circularized by performing a ligation reaction under very dilute conditions and in the presence of an excess of mutually compatible 'tag' sequence, usually in the form of a suppressor-gene construct. The circular DNA molecules are then recut with a more frequently cutting enzyme and the end fragments selectively cloned by virtue of their association with the selectable 'tag' sequence (Fig. 4.5). Now we have an easily handled lambda, cosmid, or plasmid recombinant in which the left and right halves of the insert DNA were separated on the chromosome by perhaps a megabase of DNA, so effecting a one-step 'jump' of the same magnitude. Beyond the significant technical problems associated with generating representative libraries of this type, other difficulties are apparent. Perhaps the most serious is the problem of false jumps, such that previously unlinked sequences become spuriously associated. The validity of a 'jump' must be confirmed by showing that both end-fragments map to the same chromosomal region and to an appropriately sized DNA fragment, resolved by PFGE. There is still the problem of a lack of directionality, but at least with such big 'jumps' the direction of the movement should soon be obvious.

A single 'jump' will only very rarely bridge the gap between two flanking markers. The 'jump' made by Collins *et al.* (1987) from the *MET* locus brought them 100 kbp or so closer to *CF*, but an extensive and linked series of such 'jumps' would be necessary to reach the gene. So-called 'linking' libraries are designed to solve this problem (Fig. 4.5). Here, the DNA is size-cut as for conventional library construction, but then recircularized by self-ligation rather than by ligation to vector sequences. The circular DNA is then recut with a 'rare cutter' enzyme, such as *Not* I, and the small proportion of linear DNA fragments so generated are inserted into a 'rare cutter' cloning

Molecular genetics

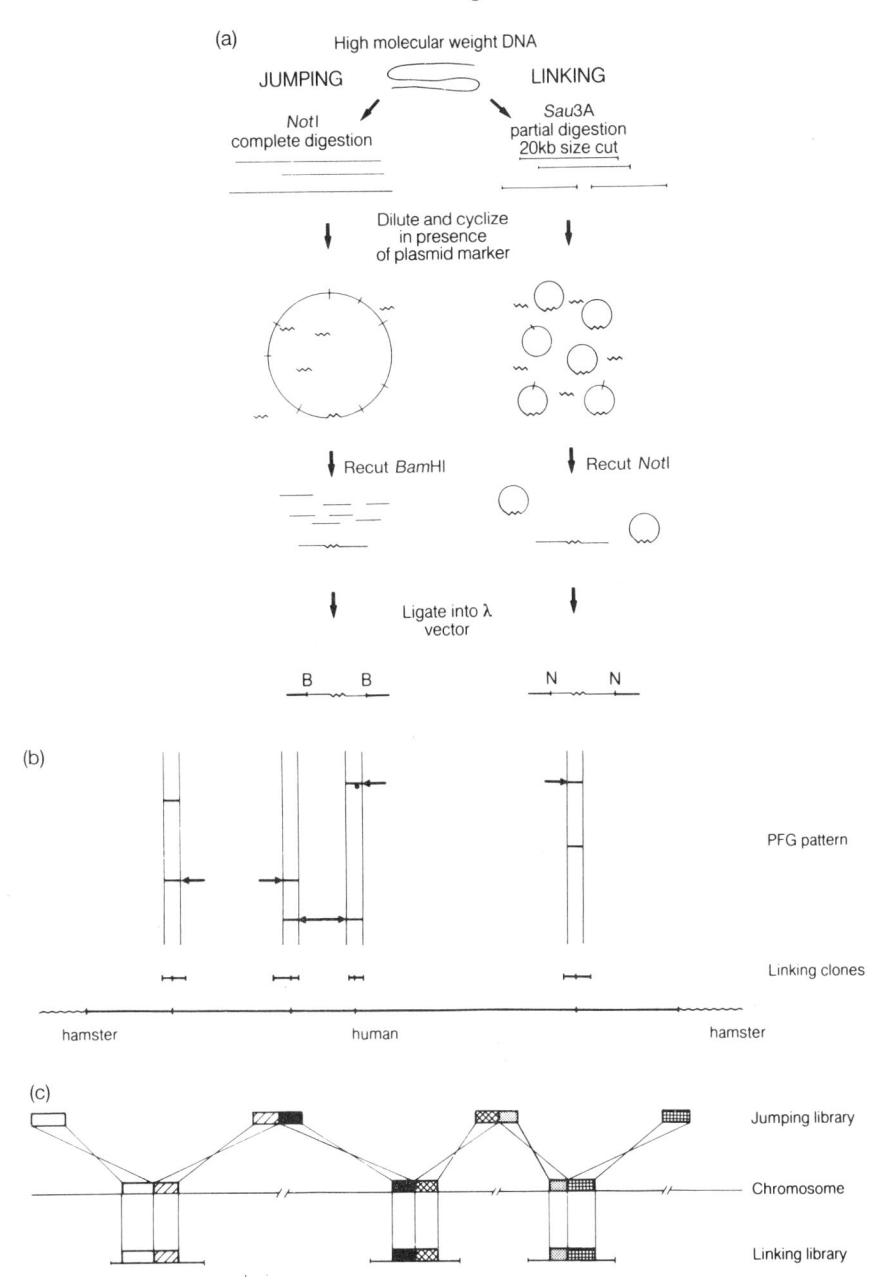

**Fig. 4.5.** The technologies of 'jumping' and 'linking' libraries. (a) Construction of the two types of library; (b) determining the order of linking probes by identifying clones hybridizing to a common restriction fragment on PFGE; (c) directional movement by alternating use of 'jumping' and 'linking' libraries (from Poustka and Lehrach 1986, with permission).

vector. Recombinants derived in this manner contain the sequences which flank either side of the genomic 'rare cutter' sites and can thus be used to 'link' adjacent, PFGE-resolved DNA fragments. Repeated isolation of cross-hybridizing 'linking' and 'jumping' clones should allow directed progress to be made along the chromosome (Fig. 4.5), as long as checks are made by PFGE analysis that each step is valid and appropriately sized.

Building up a reliable PFGE map with 'linking' and 'jumping' clones over several megabases of DNA is certainly feasible but a far from trivial task, particularily when there are no translocations or deletions interrupting the region to act as independent, confirmatory landmarks. The availability of additional DNA markers would greatly aid the map construction and tracking down the disease gene. Two methods for enrichment cloning have been tested in the search for the *CF* gene. The first again utilizes PFGE. Michels *et al.* (1987) described the isolation of a set of recombinants closely linked to *CF* by constructing a library from a *MET*-containing 450 kbp *Not* I fragment resolved by preparative PFGE. This method gave a very satisfactory 80-fold enrichment for *MET*-linked human recombinants, encouraging the extension of this strategy to new PFGE fragments now known to map closer to the *CF* locus (Estivill *et al.* 1987). However, it is important to point out that this approach is only practical if DNA is prepared from a rodent hybrid cell which contains chromosome 7 as the sole human component, so that the likelihood of more than one human fragment of the same size co-migrating on the gel is very low. This allows relevant clones from the unique human DNA fragment to be identified by their hybridization to repeated DNA sequences characteristic of human DNA and the co-purified rodent DNA recombinants to be ignored. If the starting material had been total human DNA then the vast majority of recombinants derived from *Not*I fragments co-migrating at 450 kbp would not be derived from the *MET*-containing fragment. This fact highlights the value of reduced chromosome hybrids both for mapping purposes and for enrichment cloning. Chromosome-mediated gene transfer (Porteous 1987) is one method for generating reduced chromosome hybrids and it is this approach which has made the greatest impact on the search for the *CF* gene.

## Enrichment cloning for the *CF* region following chromosome-mediated gene transfer

Chromosome-mediated gene transfer is now well established as a technique for isolating fragments of human chromosomes in mammalian cells (Porteous 1987). In brief, mitotic chromosomes are prepared from an appropriate donor cell line, co-precipitated with calcium phosphate, and applied to monolayer cultures of recipient rodent cells. Successful uptake and retention of desired chromosome fragments depends on the availability of an appropriate selection strategy for expression of a linked gene. In the case of *CF*,

Molecular genetics

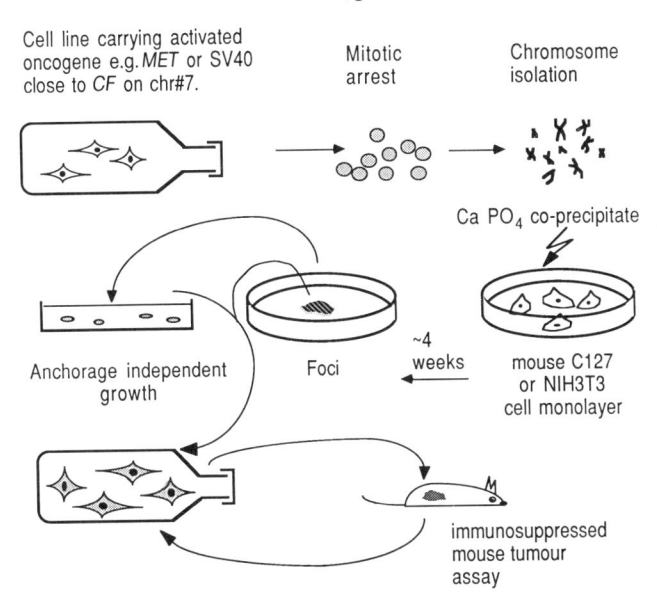

Fig. 4.6. Experimental protocol for chromosome-mediated transfection and selection for active oncogenes, either activated *MET* or the SV40 T-antigen, which map near the *CF* locus.

two complementary strategies, as outlined in Fig. 4.6, have been tested. Both utilize cellular transformation as the criterion for successful chromosomal transfer.

Our own results, using SV40-mediated cellular transformation as the co-selection for *CF*, need only brief mention. The human–mouse somatic cell hybrid Cl21 retains chromosome 7 as its sole human component. This hybrid has been used extensively in the assignment of expressed proteins and cloned DNA segments to human chromosome 7. The Cl21 hybrid is transformed by virtue of the tandem integration of SV40 genomes in chromosome 7, and we were able to show by *in situ* hybridization that the site was at band 7q31-35 (Mitchell *et al.* 1986). With *CF* localized some 5-15 Mbp centromere proximal at the 7q22/7q31 interface, CMGT for SV40 in Cl21 offered a potential co-selection strategy for *CF*. To favour expression of the *CF* gene, if co-transferred, we chose the transformation competent mouse epithelial C127 cell line, rather than NIH3T3 fibroblasts, as the chromosome recipients. Tumour-selectable foci of transformed cells gave rise to a set of transformed cells carrying variable, reduced fragments of chromosome 7 in which distant markers had been lost but *CF*-associated markers retained (unpublished results). However, these reductions in chromosome 7 complexity are accompanied by quite complex intrachromosomal rearrangements which require further characterization before evaluating their usefulness as enriched cloning resources for *CF*-linked markers. It is perhaps worth mentioning an alternative strategy (Porteous *et al.* 1987a) for generating reduced chromosome 7 hybrids without rearrangements, at least as far as can be determined at the level of preliminary PFGE analysis (unpublished). Somatic cell fusion hybrids formed between the Cl21 human precursor LNSV and mouse 3T3 cells have been reported as being non-tumorigenic (Howell 1982). However, we reasoned that if rare tumorigenic variants arose, these might be accompanied by karyotypic evolution. We were eventually able to obtain tumours following inoculation of the Cl21 cell line into immunosuppressed mice. Cytogenetic and molecular genetic analysis showed that several such tumours had undergone substantial reduction of the chromosome 7 component, but with the *CF* region apparently intact and effectively enriched several-fold. These hybrids are likely to be useful for fine-structure mapping studies around the *CF* locus. They are also ideally suited to enrichment cloning for *CF* following preparative PFGE. However, because of the considerable success already achieved with the obvious alternative CMGT approach to CF, we will concentrate and conclude by describing the efforts of the team lead by Professor R. Williamson, at St Mary's Hospital, London.

The proto-oncogene *MET* maps within a centimorgan of *CF* (see Beaudet *et al.* 1986). To date, activitation of *MET* has only been detected in the mutagenized human osteosarcoma cell line MNNG-HOS (Cooper *et al.* 1984). The activation step involves a translocation event between the 5' end of *MET* on chromosome 7 and a second locus, named *TPR* (for translocation promoter region), on chromosome 1 (Park *et al.* 1986) (see Fig. 4.7 for cytological evidence of translocation). The activation event is not simple. The parent cell line HOS carried at least two cytologically identifiable 1 : 7 translocations, neither of which appears to be transformationally active; additional MNNG-induced rearrangement at the translocation site must have taken place (Park *et al.* 1986; Tempest *et al.* 1986). Consequently, whereas the tight linkage of the *MET* proto-oncogene to *CF* demanded that MNNG-HOS be tested in CMGT, ultimate success as a strategy for cloning the *CF* gene not only required that the orientation of *MET* with respect to *CF* be compatible with co-transfer, but also that the *CF* locus had not been lost as a result of the chromosomal changes associated with *MET* activation. All of these uncertainties were additional to the inherent propensity of the CMGT process to be accompanied by intrachromosomal deletion events (Porteous *et al.* 1986; Porteous 1987). Fortunately, Williamson and colleagues were not to be put off. They established that *MET*-selected CMGT, with MNNG-HOS as chromosome donor, could indeed be used to generate hybrid cells containing as little as ~5 Mbp of DNA and retaining *D7S8* as well as *MET*, while segregating more distant markers (Scambler *et al.*

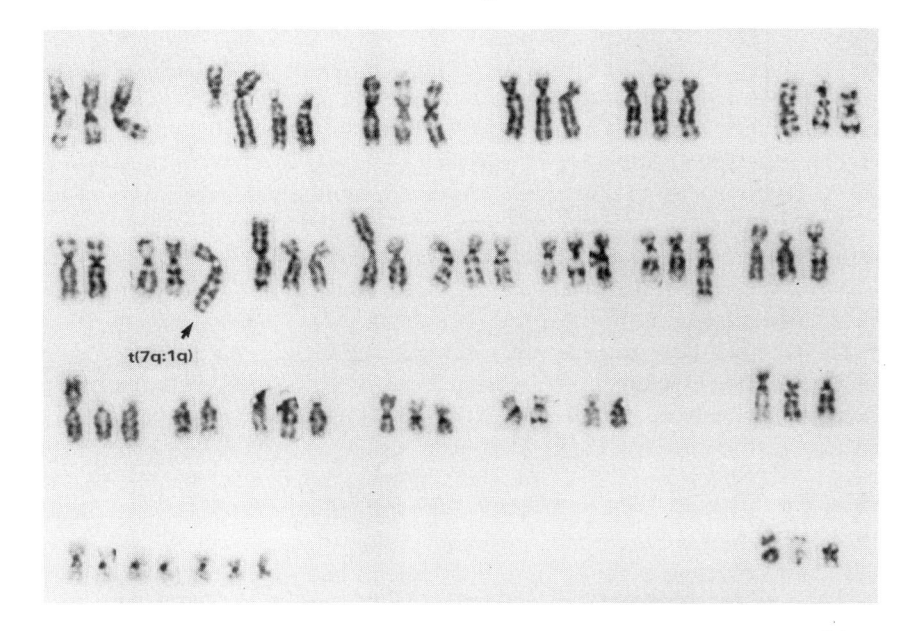

**Fig. 4.7.** A representative G-banded karyotype of the highly aneuploid cell line MNNG-HOS. The arrow indicates the 7q : 1q translocation chromosome in the chromosome 7 group. Subtle abnormalities of banding in the *MET* region can also be seen in the left-hand chromosome of this group. Similar derived chromosomes 7 are found in other MNNG-HOS sublines examined.

1986*b*). The next step was to construct genomic libraries from these reduced chromosome hybrids (Estivill *et al.* 1987), selectively isolate human recombinants, and test them for both physical and genetic linkage to *CF*. Two different strategies were used.

In the first, an extensive set of cosmid recombinants were isolated and examined for shared sequences which would indicate physical overlap and allow construction of a contiguous (hence 'contig') map of the isolated region. This aim was approached in two different ways. First, in an extension to the conventional 'walking' approach (Steinmetz *et al.* 1986), cosmids were screened for hybridization to either the *MET* or the *D7S8* probe. They were then able to 'walk' out from *D7S8* and away from *MET* along chromosome 7 and towards *CF* by using the primary cross-hybridizing cosmids to screen for newly hybridizing (and therefore distinct, but contiguous) recombinants. This procedure generated a 'contig' map of the transfectants comprising ~160 kb around *MET* and ~90 kb around *D7S8* (Scambler *et al.* 1987*b*).

Secondly, by restriction mapping randomly selected human recombinants, it was possible to recognize partially overlapping clones on the basis of shared restriction fragments. It is this procedure to which the term 'contig' mapping is more strictly applied. Success depends upon having a sufficient density of recombinants to ensure a high frequency of partial overlap. In this regard, CMGT-derived hybrids are ideal cloning resources (see also Weiss et al. 1986; Porteous et al. 1987b). However, the derived map will, of necessity, reflect the genomic configuration of the transformant, with any rearrangements of the normal which may have occurred during the CMGT process or been associated with the original donor chromosome under selection.

The second aspect of the strategy, adopted by Estivill et al. (1987), was to focus attention towards DNA sequences likely to identify genes encoding expressed functions. A genomic library was constructed in Lorist 6 (a derivative of the Lorist B cosmid cloning vector of Cross and Little (1986) ) from a *MET*-selected CMG transformant which retained only ~1 cM of human DNA, but was predicted to retain the *CF* locus. The cloning site in Lorist 6 is compatible for the restriction endonucleases *Xma* III and *Not*I, both of which occur rarely in the human genome as a whole, but are relatively enriched in the undermethylated 'islands', typically found 5' to housekeeping and some tissue-specific genes (Bird 1986; Lindsay and Bird 1987). Estivill et al. (1987) isolated two adjacent human recombinants which define a locus having many of the characteristics they were searching for. The locus *D7S23*, defined at the 5' end by the polymorphic subclone probe pCS.7, maps to the *CF* region of chromosome 7, ~700 kb from the *MET* locus. It contains an 'island' of undermethylation, rich in 'rare cutter' enzyme sites and recognizes transcripts in a variety of normal human tissues, including lung. Finally, the sub-segments defined by pCS.7, continue to segregate with *CF* in several families where recombination between *CF* and *D7S8*, or between *CF* and *MET*, was observed (Estivill et al. 1987). In addition, they show strong linkage disequilibrium (Cavalli-Sforza and Bodmer 1971) with the mutant allele at the *CF* locus. The phenomenon of linkage disequilibrium arises when specific alleles at closely linked loci are found together in one haplotype more often than expected from the allele frequencies in the general population. The very existence of strong allelic association between a tightly linked marker and a disease locus is good evidence for having arrived at, or being very near, the disease gene.

Having reached the tantalizing stage of identifying a candidate gene, arrived at so rapidly by the techniques of reverse genetics, what is left to be done before announcing with confidence that the *CF* gene has been cloned? There are several criteria which must be met before accepting a candidate as the *CF* gene:

1. Does the DNA/amino acid sequence display homology to other known genes or features consistent with the predicted function of the *CF* gene?

2. Does the gene show an expression profile consistent with our knowledge of which tissues are affected and which unaffected?
3. Is there a consistent mutational alteration in the coding or controlling sequences in affected individuals?
4. Has recombination between the disease locus and polymorphic site(s) within the candidate gene been excluded in all affected families?

In the case of this first 'reverse genetic' candidate for the *CF* gene, the answer to each of these questions must unfortunately be a tentative no (see, for example, the recombinant family described by Berger *et al.* 1987). There is sufficient doubt on points 1 and 3 above (Wainwright *et al.* 1988) to warrant a further search of nearby expressed sequences for identity with the *CF* gene. This highlights the considerable difficulty of relying so heavily upon genetic linkage to identify candidate genes, and emphasizes the enormous value of chromosomal rearrangements, either germ line or somatic, in directing the final search for an unknown disease gene (Orkin 1986). By way of compensation, there can now be little doubt that the sequence defined by pCS.7 must be within a gene or two of the *CF* locus. Perhaps it will take a sledge-hammer to crack the final nut, but this should not diminish the measure of the success of the CMGT-based approach in speeding us from a primary genetic linkage to the favourable position we are in today.

# References

Anand, R. (1986). Pulsed field gel electrophoresis: a technique for fractionating large DNA molecules. *Trends in Genetics* **2**, 278–83.

Barlow, D. P. and Lehrach, H. (1987). Genetics by gel electrophoresis: the impact of pulsed field gel electrophoresis on mammalian genetics. *Trends in Genetics* **3**, 167–71.

Beaudet, A. *et al.* (1986). Linkage of cystic fibrosis to two tightly linked DNA markers: joint report from a collaborative study. *American Journal of Human Genetics* **39**, 681–93.

Berger, W. *et al.* (1987). Crossovers in two German cystic fibrosis families determine probe order for MET 7C22 and XV-2c/CS.7. *Human Genetics* **77**, 197–9.

Bird, A. P. (1986). CpG-rich islands and the function of DNA methylation. *Nature* **321**, 209–13.

Botstein, D., White, R., Skolnick, M., and Davis, R. (1980). Construction of a genetic linkage map in man using restriction fragment length polymorphisms. *American Journal of Human Genetics* **32**, 314–31.

Bowcock, A. M. *et al.* (1986). Genetics analysis of cystic fibrosis: linkage of DNA and classical markers in multiplex families. *American Journal of Human Genetics* **39**, 699–706.

Bowman, B. H., Lockhart, L. H., and McCombs, M. L. (1969). Oyster ciliary inhibition by cystic fibrosis factor. *Science* **165**, 325–6.

Brock, D.J.H., Hayward, C., and Super, M. (1982). Controlled trial of serum isoelectric focussing of the cystic fibrosis gene. *Human Genetics* **60**, 30–1.

Cavalli-Sforza, L.L. and Bodmer, W.F. (1971). *The genetics of human populations.* W.H. Freeman, San Francisco.

Collins, F.S., Drumm, M.L., Cole, J.L., Lockwood, W.K., Vande Woude, G.F., and Jannuzzi, M.C. (1987). Construction of a general human chromosome jumping library, with application to cystic fibrosis. *Science* **235**, 1046–9.

Conover, J.H. *et al.* (1973). Studies on ciliary dyskinesia factor in cystic fibrosis. I. Bioassay and heterozygote detection in serum. *Pediatric Research* **7**, 220–3.

Conover, J.H., Conod, E.J., and Hirschhorn, K. (1974). Studies on ciliary dyskinesia factor in cystic fibrosis: IV, its possible identification as anaphylatoxin (C3a)-IgG complex. *Life Sciences* **14**, 253–6.

Cooper, C.S. *et al.* (1984). Molecular cloning of a new transforming gene from a chemically transformed human cell line. *Nature* **311**, 29–33.

Cross, S.H. and Little, P.F.R. (1986). A cosmid vector for systematic chromosome walking. *Gene* **49**, 9–22.

Davies, K.E., Gilliam, T.C., and Williamson, R. (1983). Cystic fibrosis is not caused by a defect in the gene coding for human complement C3. *Molecular Biology and Medicine* **1**, 185–90.

Dorin, J.R., Novak, M., Hill, R.E., Brock, D.J..H., Secher, D.S., and van Heyningen, V. (1987). A clue to the basic defect in cystic fibrosis from cloning the CF antigen gene. *Nature* **326**, 614–17.

Drumm, M.L., Smith C.L., Dean, M., Cole, J.L., Iannuzzi, M.C., and Collins, F.S. (1988). Physical mapping of the cystic fibrosis region by pulsed-field gel electrophoresis. *Genomics* **2**, 346–54.

Eiberg, H. *et al.* (1985a). Cystic fibrosis, linkage with PON. *Cytongenetics and Cell Genetics* **40**, 623.

Eiberg, H., Schmiegelow, K., Nielsen, L.S., and Williamson, R. (1985b). Linkage relationships of paraoxonase (PON) with other markers: indication of PON-cystic fibrosis synteny. *Clinical Genetics* **28**, 265–71.

Estivill, X., Schmidtke, J., Williamson, R., and Wainwright, B. (1986). Chromosome assignment and restriction fragment length polymorphism analysis of the anonymous DNA probe B79a at 7q22. *Human Genetics* **74**, 320–2.

Estivill, X. *et al.* (1987). A candidate for the cystic fibrosis locus isolated by selection for methylation-free islands. *Nature* **326**, 840–5.

Farrall, M. *et al.* (1986a). First-trimester prenatal diagnosis of cystic fibrosis with linked DNA probes. *Lancet* **i**, 1402–5.

Farrall, M. *et al.* (1986b). Cystic fibrosis carrier detection using a linked gene probe. *Journal of Medical Genetics* **23**, 295–9.

Forrest, S.M., Cross, G.S., Speer, A., Gardner-Medwin, D., Burn, J., and Davies, K.E. (1987). Preferential deletion of exons in Duchenne and Becker muscular dystrophies. *Nature* **329**, 638–40.

Frizzel, R.A., Rechkemmer, F., and Shoemaker, R.L. (1986). Altered regulation of airway epithelial cell chloride channels in cystic fibrosis. *Science* **233**, 558–60.

Graham, J.B., Barrow, E.S., Reisner, H.M., and Edgell, C-J. (1983). The genetics of blood coagulation. *Advances in Human Genetics* **13**, 1–81.

Grataroli, R., Guy-Crotte, O., Galabert, C., and Figarella, C. (1984). Detection of cystic fibrosis protein by isoelectric focusing of serum and plasma. *Pediatric Research* **18**, 130-3.
Harris, H. (1980). *Principles of human biochemical genetics*, (3rd edn). Elsevier North Holland, Amsterdam.
Hashem, N. *et al.* (1980). Clinical characteristics, DNA repair and complementation groups in xeroderma pigmentosum patients from Egypt. *Cancer Research* **40**, 13-18.
Hayward, C., Glass, S., van Heyningen, V., and Brock, D.J.H. (1987). Serum concentrations of a granulocyte-derived calcium-binding protein in cystic fibrosis patient and heterozygotes. *Clinical Chimica Acta* **170**, 45-56.
Howell, N. (1982). Suppression of transformation and tumorigenicity in interspecies hybrids of human SV40-transformed and mouse 3T3 cell lines. *Cytogenetics and Cell Genetics* **34**, 215-29.
Hulten, M. (1974). Chiasma distribution at diakinesis in the normal human male. *Hereditas* **76**, 55-78.
Human gene mapping, 8 (1985). *Cytogenetics and Cell Genetics* **40**, 1-823.
Knowlton, R.G. *et al.* (1985). A polymorphic DNA marker linked to cystic fibrosis is located on chromosome 7. *Nature* **318**, 380-2.
Lindsay, S. and Bird, A.P. (1987). Use of restriction enzymes to detect potential gene sequences in mammalian DNA. *Nature* **327**, 336-8.
McKusick, V.A. (1986). *Mendelian inheritance in man*, (7th edn). Johns Hopkins University Press, Baltimore.
Manson, J.C. and Brock, D.J.H. (1980). Development of a quantitative immunoassay for the cystic fibrosis gene. *Lancet* **i**, 330-1.
Mayo, B.J., Klebe, R.J., Barnett, D.R., Lankford, B.J., and Bowman, B.H. (1980). Somatic cell genetic studies of the cystic fibrosis mucociliary inhibitor. *Clinical Genetics* **18**, 379-86.
Michiels, F., Burmeister, M., and Lehrach, H. (1987). Derivation of clones close to *met* by preparative field inversion gel electorphoresis. *Science* **236**, 1305-8.
Mitchell, A.R., Ambros, P., Gosden, J.R., Morten, J.E.N., and Porteous, D.J. (1986). Gene mapping and physical arrangements of human chromatin in transformed hybrid cells: fluorescent and autoradiographic *in situ* hybridization compared. *Somatic Cell and Molecular Genetics* **12**, 313-24.
Neufeld, E.F. and Fratantoni, J.C. (1970). Inborn errors of mucopoly saccharide metabolism. Faulty degradative mechanisms are implicated in this group of human diseases. *Science* **169**, 141-6.
Nevin, G.B., Nevin, N.C., Redmond, A.O., Young, I.R., and Tully, W.G. (1981). Detection of cystic fibrosis homozygotes and heterozygotes by serum isoelectric focusing. *Human Genetics* **56**, 387-9.
Orkin, S.H. (1986). Reverse genetics and human disease. *Cell* **47**, 845-50.
Palumbo, A.P. *et al.* (1986). Chromosomal localisation of a human band 3-like gene to region 7q35→7q36. *American Journal of Human Genetics* **39**, 307-16.
Park, M. *et al.* (1986). Mechanism of *met* oncogene activation. *Cell* **45**, 895-904.
Porteous, D.J. (1987). Chromosome mediated gene transfer: a functional assay for complex loci and an aid to human genome mapping. *Trends in Genetics* **3**, 177-182.

Porteous, D. J. and van Heyningen, V. (1986). Cystic fibrosis: from linked markers to the gene. *Trends in Genetics* **2**, 149-52.

Porteous, D. J. *et al*. (1986). Molecular and physical arrangements of human DNA in *HRASI*-selected, chromosome-mediated transfectants. *Molecular and Cellular Biology* **6**, 2223-32.

Porteous, D.J., Wilkinson, M., Fletcher, J., and van Heyningen, V. (1987a). Tumour growth selects hybrids carrying fragments of single human chromosomes. Human gene mapping 9. *Cytogenetics and Cell Genetics* **46**, 677.

Porteous, D.J. *et al* (1987b). HRASI-selected chromosome transfer generates markers that colocalize anirida- and genitourinary dysplasia-associated translocation breakpoints and the Wilms' tumor gene within band 11p13. *Proceedings of the National Academy of Sciences* **84**, 5355-9.

Poustka, A.M. and Lehrach, H. (1986). Jumping libraries and linking libraries: the next generation of molecular tools in mammalian genetics. *Trends in Genetics* **2**, 174-9.

Poustka, A.M.., Lehrach, H., Williamson, R., and Bates, G. (1988). A long range restriction map encompassing the cystic fibrosis locus and its closely linked genetic markers. *Genomics* **2**, 337-45.

Renwick, J.H. (1969). Progress in mapping human autosomes. *British Medical Bulletin* **25**, 65-73.

Romeo, G. *et al*. (1985). Incidence in Italy, genetic heterogeneity and segregation analysis of cystic fibrosis. *American Journal of Human Genetics* **37**, 338-49.

Scambler, P. *et al*. (1985). Linkage studies between polymorphic markers on chromosome 4 and cystic fibrosis. *Human Genetics* **69**, 250-4.

Scambler, P.J., Wainwright, B.J., Watson, E., Bell, G., Williamson, R., and Farrall, M. (1986a). Isolation of a further anonymous informative DNA sequence from chromosome seven closely linked to cystic fibrosis. *Nucleic Acids Research* **14**, 1951-6.

Scambler, P.J., Law, H-Y., Williamson, R., and Cooper, C.S. (1986b). Chromosome mediated gene transfer of six DNA markers linked to the cystic fibrosis locus on human chromosome 7. *Nucleic Acids Research* **14**, 7159-174.

Scambler, P.J., McPherson, M.A., Bates, G., Bradbury, N.A., Dormer, R.L., and Williamson, R. (1987a). Biochemical and genetic exclusion of calmodulin as the site of the basic defect in cystic fibrosis. *Human Genetics* **76**, 278-82.

Scambler, P.J. *et al*. (1987b). Physical and genetic analysis of cosmids from the vicinity of the cystic fibrosis locus. *Nucleic Acids Research* **15**, 3639-52.

Schmidtke, J. *et al*. (1987). Linkage relationships and allelic associations of the cystic fibrosis locus and four marker loci. *Human Genetics* **76**, 337-43.

Schwartz, D.C. and Cantor, C.R. (1984). Separation of yeast chromosome-sized DNAs by pulsed field gradient gel electrophoresis. *Cell* **37**, 67-75.

Sing, C.F., Risser, D.R., Howatt, W.F., and Erickson, R.P. (1982). Phenotypic heterogeneity in cystic fibrosis. *American Journal of Medical Genetics*. **13**, 179-195.

Solomon, E., and Bodmer, W.F. (1979). Evolution of the sickle variant gene. *Lancet* **i**, 923.

Steinmetz, M., Stephan, D., and Fisher-Lindahl, K. (1986). Gene organization and recombinational hotspots in the murine major histocompatibility complex. *Cell* **44**, 895-904.

Talamo, R. C., Rosenstein, B. J., and Berninger, R. W. (1983). Cystic fibrosis. In *The metabolic basis of inherited disease*, (5th edn), (ed. J. B. Stanbury, J. B. Wyngaarden, D. S. Fredrickson, J. L. Goldstein, and M. S. Brown). McGraw Hill, New York.

Tempest, P. R., Reeves, B. R., Spurr, N. K., Rance, A. J., Chan, A. M-L., and Brookes, P. (1986). Activation of the *met* oncogene in the human MNNG-HOS cell line involves a chromosomal rearrangement. *Carcinogenesis* 7, 2051-7.

Tsui, L-C. *et al.* (1985). Cystic fibrosis locus defined by a genetically linked polymorphic DNA marker. *Science* 230, 1054-7.

van Heyningen, V., Hayward, C., Fletcher, J., and McAuley, C. (1985*a*). Tissue localization and chromosomal assignment of a serum protein that tracks the cystic fibrosis gene. *Nature* 315, 513-15.

van Heyningen, V., *et al.* (1985*b*). Molecular analysis of chromosome 11 deletions in aniridia-Wilms' tumor syndrome. *Proceedings of the National Academy of Sciences* 82, 8592-6.

van Heyningen, V. and Porteous, D. J. (1986). Mapping a chromosome to find a gene. *Trends in Genetics* 2, 4-5.

Wainwright, B. J. *et al.* (1985). Localization of cystic fibrosis locus to human chromosome 7cen-q22. *Nature* 318 384-5.

Wainwright, B. J., Scambler, P. J., and Williamson, R. (1987). Regional localization of three probes closely linked to the cystic fibrosis locus by deletion analysis. *Cytogenetics and Cell Genetics* 44, 101-2.

Wainwright, B. J. *et al.* (1988). Isolation of a human gene with protein sequence similarity to human and murine *int-1* and the *Drosophila* segment polarity mutant *wingless*. *EMBO Journal* 7, 1743-8.

Weatherall, D. J. (1985). *The new genetics and clinical practice*, (2nd edn). Oxford University Press.

Weiss, J. H., Seidman, J. G., Housman, D. E., and Nelson, D. L. (1986). Eucaryotic chromosome transfer: production of a murine-specific cosmid library from a neo-linked fragment of murine chromosome 17. *Molecular and Cellular Biology* 6, 441-51.

Welsh, M. J. and Liedtke, C. M. (1986). Chloride and potassium channels in cystic fibrosis airway epithelia. *Nature* 322, 467-70.

White, R. *et al.* (1985*a*). Construction of linkage maps with DNA markers for human chromosomes. *Nature* 313, 101-5.

White, R. *et al.* (1985*b*). A closely linked genetic marker for cystic fibrosis. *Nature* 318, 382-4.

Wilson, G. B., Fudenberg, H. H., and Jahn, T. L. (1975). Studies on cystic fibrosis using isoelectric focusing. I. An assay for detection of cystic fibrosis homozygotes and heterozygote carriers from serum. *Pediatric Research* 9, 635-40.

Wright, A. F. (1986). DNA analysis in human disease. *Journal of Clinical Pathology* 39, 1281-95.

Zengerling, S., Olek, K., Tsui, L.-C., Grzeschik, K.-H., Riordan, J. R., and Buchwald, M. (1987). Mapping of DNA markers linked to the cystic fibrosis locus on the long arm of chromosome 7. *American Journal of Human Genetics* 40, 228-36.

# 5 Prenatal diagnosis
DAVID J.H. BROCK

## Introduction

The traditional method of diagnosing genetic disorders *in utero* is by measuring the protein product of the mutant gene in an accessible fetal tissue. For cystic fibrosis (CF) prenatal diagnosis in this way is not yet an option. Although the chromosomal localization of the *CF* gene is known (see Chapter 4), and although there are suggestions that the gene itself may have been identified (Estivill *et al.* 1987a), the nature of the protein product has not yet been ascertained. For the present, therefore, methods of prenatal diagnosis must necessarily remain indirect.

Nonetheless, successful *in utero* detection of CF fetuses has been a part of specialized antenatal care for several years. One method depends on monitoring early clinical signs of the disorder by measurement of a group of microvillar enzymes in second-trimester amniotic fluid samples. The other exploits the tight linkage of an arbitrary set of DNA markers to the *CF* gene, and can be applied either to chorionic villus samples (CVS) taken in the first or second trimester of pregnancy, or to second-trimester amniotic fluid cells. Each method has its own advantages and disadvantages. It is to be hoped that both will become obsolete as the detailed molecular biology of CF unravels.

## The risk of having a child with cystic fibrosis

There have been many suggestions in the past, based on the clinical heterogeneity of the disorder, that CF might be several distinct diseases masquerading under the same name. There now seems little doubt that, at least amongst people of Caucasian origin, CF is a genetically homogeneous entity. The discovery of DNA markers tightly linked to the *CF* gene has allowed the chromosomal locus to be mapped to a specific region of the long arm of chromosome 7; 7q21–q31 (Knowlton *et al.* 1985; Tsui *et al.* 1985; Wainwright *et al.* 1985; White *et al.* 1985). A large collaborative survey of families collected from Europe and North America (Beaudet *et al.* 1986) showed that in all informative cases the *CF* gene was linked to chromosome 7 markers, and therefore in all probability coded for by the same genetic locus. More recent linkage information has gone further and suggested that a majority of North European CF families have inherited the same mutant allele from their ancestors (Estivill *et al*. 1987*a*). If this is the case, CF may turn out to have a formal similarity to sickle-cell anaemia—a genetic disorder caused by a very limited number of mutational events, all at one genetic locus.

From the point of view of genetic counselling, the estimation of risk is based on observations that CF is inherited as a typical Mendelian recessive. The most frequently encountered situation where prenatal diagnosis is requested is for the couple who have already had one or more children affected with CF. As in all conditions inherited as autosomal recessives, the recurrence risk is 1 in 4 and does not change in successive pregnancies whatever the previous outcome. There is a tantalizing suggestion (Boué *et al*. 1986) that if the index affected child has meconium ileus, the recurrence risk for any form of CF may be greater than the theoretical expectation of 25 per cent. However, since the numbers on which this observation is based are small, and since it does not accord with any reasonable model for the genetics of the disorder, it should be viewed with considerable caution.

If a couple present, each of whom has a sibling with CF, their risk of conceiving an affected child is 1 in 9. This follows from the fact that the normal siblings of CF homozygotes have a two-thirds chance of being heterozygotes, and a one-third chance of passing the gene to their offspring in each pregnancy (Fig. 5.1).

If, on the other hand, both husband and wife have siblings who have borne affected children, the couple's risk of conceiving an affected child is 1 in 16. This arises because the sibling of an obligate heterozygote has a half chance of also being a heterozygote and a one-quarter chance of passing the gene to his or her offspring (Fig. 5.1).

The risks of recurrence and occurrence shown in Fig. 5.1 are independent of the gene frequency. For the pedigrees shown in Fig. 5.2 it is assumed that the incidence of CF is 1 in 2500, that the gene frequency is therefore 0.02 (1 in 50), and the heterozygote frequency 0.04 (1 in 25). The calculations in Fig. 5.2 assume that CF is governed by a single genetic locus, but can accommodate different mutant alleles provided each is fully penetrant.

## DNA-based methods of prenatal diagnosis

Over the past decade a number of new laboratory techniques have been developed for the manipulation and analysis of DNA. They may be applied to any tissues which contain nucleated cells and can thus be used to detect or track mutant genes in tissues in which the gene product is either not expressed or where the question of expression remains uncertain. For the purposes of prenatal diagnosis both CVS or cultured amniotic fluid cells provide adequate amounts of genomic DNA. In a chorionic biopsy the expected yield

Couple has one (or more) affected child(ren)                    RISK

1/2 x 1/2        1 in 4

Wife and husband both have affected sibs

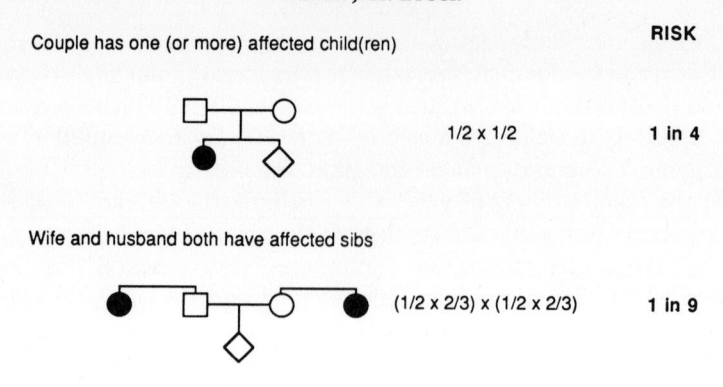

(1/2 x 2/3) x (1/2 x 2/3)       1 in 9

Wife and husband both have carrier sibs

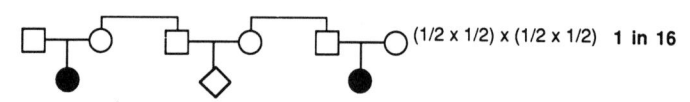

(1/2 x 1/2) x (1/2 x 1/2)   1 in 16

**Fig. 5.1.** Recurrence and occurrence risks in CF families.

of isolated DNA is about 0.1 per cent or 1 $\mu$g per mg wet weight of tissue. Cultured amniotic fluid cells yield about 100 $\mu$g of DNA per $10^8$ cells, and this amount of material can be accumulated after 10–14 days of laboratory culture.

Prenatal diagnosis is most powerful when DNA probes are available that directly recognize the disease mutation present in a specific family (Wilson et al. 1982; Kidd et al. 1983). This ideal situation can only be achieved when the gene causing the disease has been cloned and the molecular basis of the disease has been determined. In the absence of probes for the CF gene, prenatal diagnosis can be achieved by linkage analysis.

Although linkage analysis has been used for many years in the diagnosis of genetic diseases, its power has been greatly enhanced in recent years by the discoveries of molecular biology. Two factors have contributed to these advances. The first is the availability of large numbers of cloned DNA fragments, sometimes representing actual genes and sometimes 'anonymous' fragments, which can be used as markers of disease genes.

The second factor is one which could not have been predicted 10 years ago. Throughout the human genome there is a great deal of variation in individual base pairs making up the DNA, much of it occurring in regions which do not encode specific messenger RNA or carry regulatory sequences. This variation appears to have no discernible effect on the phenotype and is referred to as neutral mutation or polymorphism. Many of these neutral

## Prenatal diagnosis

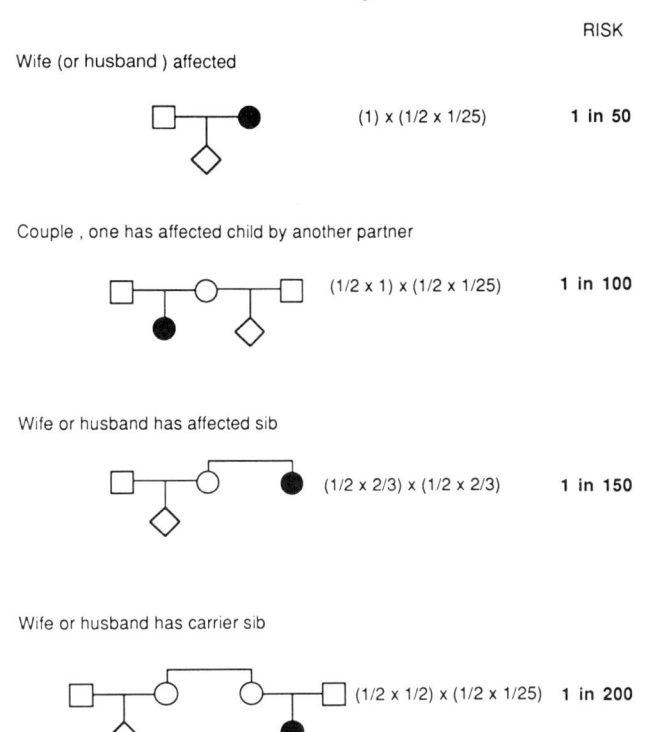

Wife (or husband) affected

(1) x (1/2 x 1/25)    RISK: **1 in 50**

Couple, one has affected child by another partner

(1/2 x 1) x (1/2 x 1/25)    **1 in 100**

Wife or husband has affected sib

(1/2 x 2/3) x (1/2 x 2/3)    **1 in 150**

Wife or husband has carrier sib

(1/2 x 1/2) x (1/2 x 1/25)    **1 in 200**

**Fig. 5.2.** Occurrence risks for CF if the gene frequency is 0.02.

mutations alter existing restriction enzyme recognition sites, either by abolishing them or by introducing new ones. Thus, digestion of genomic DNA from two different individuals with a battery of restriction enzymes will always produce a set of DNA fragments which are individual-specific. However, recognition of the variation in fragments depends on having an appropriate probe.

When a suitable probe is available it can be used to follow mutation in a restriction site on a Southern blot. If mutation has abolished the site, the resulting fragment will be larger and will travel less far in the agarose gel electrophoresis which precedes blotting (Southern 1975). Conversely, if a new recognition site has been introduced, a smaller fragment will run further on the gel and be identified towards the anodic end.

Since the variation revealed by restriction enzymes is in the size or length of the fragments, they are known as restriction fragment length polymorphisms, or RFLPs. We must note that since humans are diploid organisms, individuals can be either homozygous or heterozygous for a particular RFLP.

When an RFLP is found to be linked to a particular disease gene, it can be used to track the gene through several generations of a family. However, it is not usually known in advance which of the two (or more) polymorphic variants segregates with the disease gene and which segregates with the normal gene. Thus, in any form of linkage analysis (or indirect gene analysis) establishing the phase relationship of gene and marker is of critical importance.

# Prenatal diagnosis of cystic fibrosis by linkage analysis

## Probes suitable for CF detection

In November 1985 a number of papers appeared describing RFLPs linked to the *CF* gene. This was the culmination of a long and systematic search for linkage, involving collaboration between several laboratories in screening large CF families against a battery of markers. The current map of the *CF* locus is shown in Chapter 4. From the point of view of this chapter, the markers that matter are defined by the tightly linked probes pJ3.11 (*D7S8*), pmet H (*MET*), pmet D (*MET*), p7C22 (*D7S18*) and p79a (*D7S13*) (Wainwright *et al.* 1985; White *et al.* 1985; Estivill *et al.* 1986; Scambler *et al.* 1986). Limited data are also available on the more recently isolated probes pXV-2c and pCS.7 which define the locus *D7S23* (Estivill *et al.* 1987*a*).

Each of the above probes defines at least one polymorphism with two alleles. As shown in Table 5.1, selection of suitable restriction enzymes can reveal more than one polymorphism with pJ3.11, pmet H, pmet D, and p79a. However, in some of the polymorphisms the major allele occurs so frequently

Table 5.1. DNA probes for use in prenatal diagnosis of CF

| Probe | Restriction enzyme | No. of alleles | Size of alleles (kbp) | Frequency of major allele |
|---|---|---|---|---|
| pJ3.11 | *Msp*I | 2 | 4.2/1.8 | 0.5 |
|  | *Taq*I | 2 | 6.3/3.1 | 0.95 |
| pmet H | *Msp*I | 3 | 5.0/2.3/1.8 | 0.6 |
|  | *Taq*I | 2 | 7.5/4.0 | 0.7 |
| pmet D | *Taq*I | 2 | 6.0/4.4 | 0.85 |
|  | *Ban*I | 2 | 7.6/6.8 | 0.6 |
| p7C22 | *Eco*RI | 2 | 7. 2/5.1 | 0.75 |
| p79a | *Msp*I | 2 | 11.6/8.4 | 0.6 |
|  | *Hind*III | 2 | 8.1/4.3 | 0.7 |
| pXV-2c | *Taq*1 | 2 | 2.1/1.4 | 0.5 |
| pCS.7 | *Hha*I | 2 | 0.7/0.5 | 0.6 |

(for example, pJ3.11 with *Taq*I) that the chances of any individual being heterozygous for both alleles (and therefore informative) is quite low.

Because each of the RFLPs in Table 5.1 is defined by a site very close to the *CF* gene, they can be regarded as a set of nearly independent markers giving relevant information on the segregation of the disease. Normal practice is to type a family first with the most favoured probe and enzyme, and then to work through the other markers according to custom and experience, until segregation is fully informative (see below). It is most unusual to find a family where even one parent is homozygous for each RFLP. However, because some alleles associate with each other more often than would be expected by chance (a phenomenon known as linkage disequilibrium), the markers are not truly independent, and one can occasionally find families where one or other parent is not informative.

## Phase and informativeness

The first step in the application of RFLPs to prenatal diagnosis of CF is to establish the phase relationship between the markers and the *CF* gene. In most situations this is effected by examining bands on Southern blots of DNA taken from the blood of both parents and from the index affected child. If the affected child is no longer alive, or is not available for typing, it is normally not possible to proceed with this form of diagnosis (but see below).

Consider, for example, the phase relationships shown in Fig. 5.3. Here we are considering only a single DNA marker with two alleles, for convenience called $A_1$ and $A_2$. In the top pedigree, each of the parents is heterozygous for this marker while the index affected child is homozygous for the $A_2$ allele. This means that we have a fully informative pregnancy. If a CVS is obtained from the at-risk pregnancy at eight or nine weeks of gestation and a Southern blot shows an $A_2A_2$ band pattern, it indicates that the fetus is affected with CF. If the band pattern is either $A_1A_2$ or $A_1A_1$, the fetus is unaffected; the former indicating a CF heterozygote and the latter a homozygous normal.

In the lower pedigree in Fig. 5.3, the at-risk pregnancy is only partially informative. This follows from the fact that the index affected child has the same heterozygous band pattern as each of its parents. The *CF* gene may be linked to either the $A_1$ or $A_2$ allele in the father and to either the $A_2$ or $A_1$ allele in the mother. Without further information from other markers, one cannot distinguish between these two possibilities. Thus an $A_1A_2$ band pattern in the at-risk CVS can indicate either an affected infant or a homozygous normal. On the other hand, an $A_1A_1$ band pattern or an $A_2A_2$ band pattern signals an unaffected fetus.

Fortunately, the above information can be known before the CVS is taken. Parents can be counselled that the at-risk pregnancy is only partially informative and that they have only a 50 per cent chance of getting a definitive answer. If they do decide to proceed with first-trimester prenatal

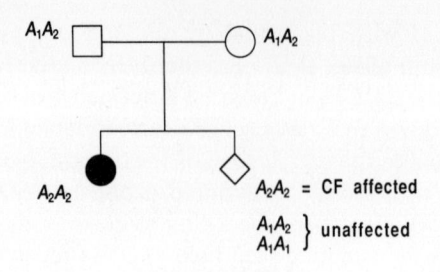

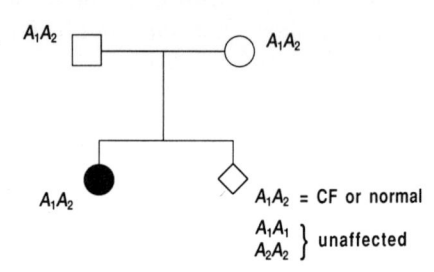

## Fig. 5.3. Illustration of fully and partially informative pregnancies.

Top pedigree:
- Father: $A_1A_2$, Mother: $A_1A_2$
- Affected daughter: $A_2A_2$
- Fetus (CVS): $A_2A_2$ = CF affected; $A_1A_2$ or $A_1A_1$ = unaffected

Bottom pedigree:
- Father: $A_1A_2$, Mother: $A_1A_2$
- Affected daughter: $A_1A_2$
- Fetus (CVS): $A_1A_2$ = CF or normal; $A_1A_1$ or $A_2A_2$ = unaffected

diagnosis, and if the band pattern in the CVS turns out to be $A_1A_2$, they will know that the mother is carrying a fetus with a 50 per cent risk of CF. They may decide to opt for termination of pregnancy or to proceed to a second-trimester amniocentesis in the hope that the uncertainty about prognosis will be revealed at that time.

The availability of several DNA probes tightly linked to the *CF* gene means that a large proportion of at-risk pregnancies can be rendered fully informative. This is illustrated schematically in Fig. 5.4. Here the probe pJ3.11 has been used in combination with the restriction endonuclease *Msp*I, and the probe pmet H in combination with endonuclease *Taq*I. The actual band patterns seen on two different Southern blots have been combined and are shown below the different individuals within the pedigree. Note that neither probe is on its own fully informative. If only pJ3.11 were used, it would not be possible to distinguish between the affected index child and its mother. If only pmet H were used, the affected child would have the same band pattern as its father. However, when the results of both Southern blots are combined, a unique pattern is seen for the index child. Of the four possible combinations of band patterns which might be seen in the CVS, only one is the same as that in the index child, and this would signal unambiguously that we are dealing with an affected fetus.

Unravelling the band patterns on Southern blots and assigning genotypes is

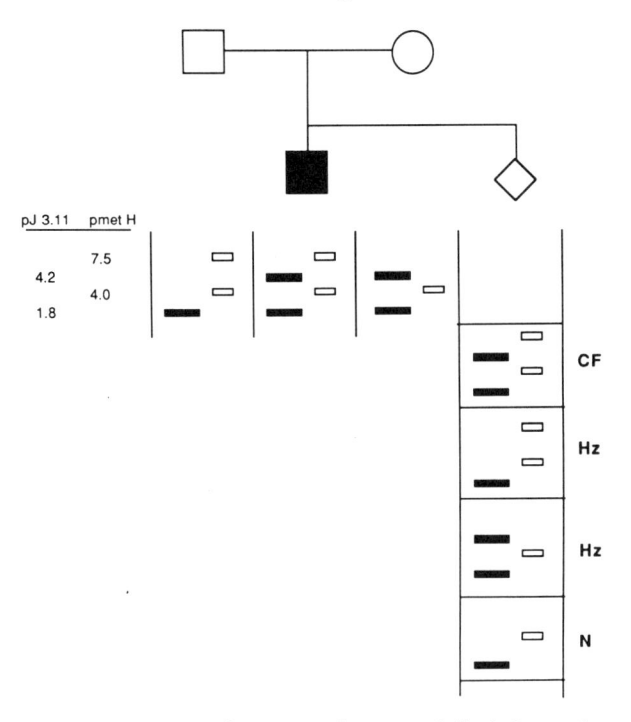

**Fig. 5.4.** Use of two DNA markers to make a partially informative pregnancy fully informative.

not immediately obvious, even to the specialist. The normal way of dealing with the situation outlined in Fig. 5.4 is to start with the index affected child and consider the possible phase relationships. As shown in Fig. 5.5, there are at first sight two possibilities. Since the affected child must have inherited a *CF* allele from each parent, it can either have the chromosomes indicated in A or those indicated in B. In A the *1.8 kbp pj3.11* allele is in phase with the *7.5 kbp pmet H* allele, while in B the phase relationship is reversed. Inspection of the band patterns in the father shows that his contribution to the affected child must have been the *7.5 kbp pmet H* allele (since the mother does not have this allele) and that therefore his 'CF' chromosome must have the *1.8 kbp pj3.11* allele in phase with the *7.5 kbp pmet H* allele. In turn, inspection of the phase relationships in the mother—who has a unique *4.2 kbp pj3.11* allele—shows that her 'CF' chromosome must have the *4.2 kbp pj3.11 allele* in phase with the *4.0 kbp pmet H* allele. This establishes the phase relationships in the index affected child (A) and in the father (C) and mother (E). We can therefore outline the four possible combinations of chromosomes in putative offspring (Fig. 5.5) and note that each gives unique information on the genotype of the fetus.

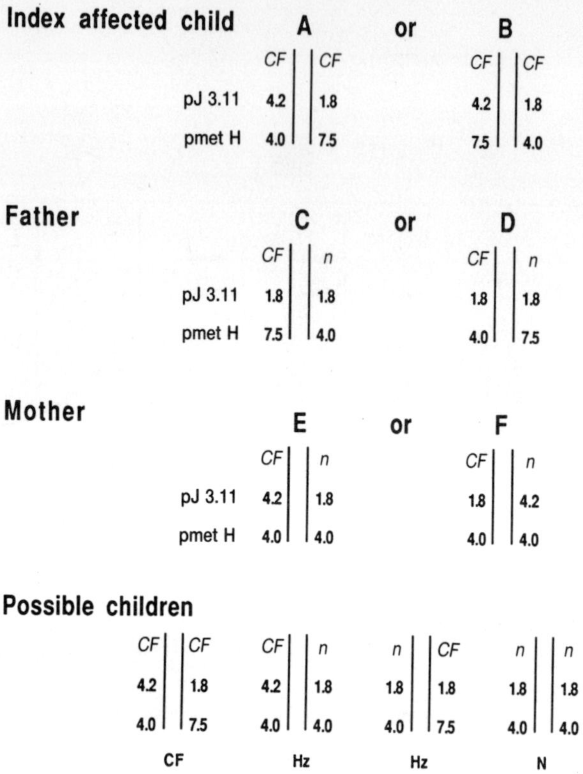

**Index affected child**

|  | A |  | or | B |  |
|---|---|---|---|---|---|
|  | CF | CF |  | CF | CF |
| pJ 3.11 | 4.2 | 1.8 |  | 4.2 | 1.8 |
| pmet H | 4.0 | 7.5 |  | 7.5 | 4.0 |

**Father**

|  | C |  | or | D |  |
|---|---|---|---|---|---|
|  | CF | n |  | CF | n |
| pJ 3.11 | 1.8 | 1.8 |  | 1.8 | 1.8 |
| pmet H | 7.5 | 4.0 |  | 4.0 | 7.5 |

**Mother**

|  | E |  | or | F |  |
|---|---|---|---|---|---|
|  | CF | n |  | CF | n |
| pJ 3.11 | 4.2 | 1.8 |  | 1.8 | 4.2 |
| pmet H | 4.0 | 4.0 |  | 4.0 | 4.0 |

**Possible children**

| CF | CF | CF | n | n | CF | n | n |
|---|---|---|---|---|---|---|---|
| 4.2 | 1.8 | 4.2 | 1.8 | 1.8 | 1.8 | 1.8 | 1.8 |
| 4.0 | 7.5 | 4.0 | 4.0 | 4.0 | 7.5 | 4.0 | 4.0 |
| CF |  | Hz |  | Hz |  | N |  |

**Fig. 5.5.** Unravelling phase relationships.

## No index affected child

In general, it is difficult to perform prenatal diagnosis within a nuclear family unless there is an index affected child to establish phase relationships. Even when unaffected children are available for typing, one does not know whether they are homozygous normals or heterozygous normals. This is illustrated in Fig. 5.6a. Here, the index affected child has died before typing was possible. The genotype of the unaffected child shows that the maternal chromosome contains a *1.8 kbp pj3.11* allele and a *7.5 kbp pmet H* allele, or in other words a *1.8/7.5* haplotype. The paternal chromosome must therefore have a *4.2/7.5* haplotype. However, we do not know whether either or neither of these haplotypes is in linkage with a *CF* allele. (It cannot be both, since the child is unaffected). Thus, the only genotype in a CVS in which we can exclude homozygosity for the *CF* gene is that identical to the unaffected child. Other genotypes would be ambiguous.

This uncertainty can sometimes be resolved if there is an extended family

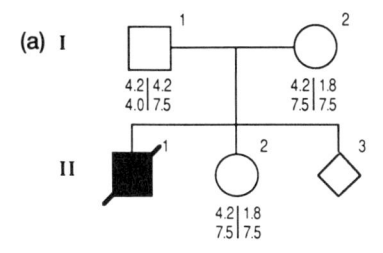

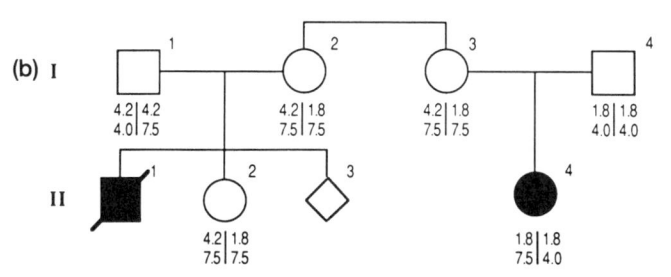

**Fig. 5.6.** Phase relationships cannot be established when the index affected child is dead (a), unless there is an affected infant elsewhere in the family (b).

from which phase relationships can be inferred. In Fig. 5.6b, the mother's sister (I-3) must also be a carrier of the *CF* gene, since she has an affected child (II-4). Inspection of the genotype of the affected child shows that the *CF* allele on the maternal side of the family must be in linkage with the *1.8/7.5* haplotype. Since the unaffected child (II-2) has inherited this haplotype, its normality must be ensured by getting a *4.2/7.5* haplotype with a normal gene from its father. In this way we have established the phase relationship within the nuclear family and such a pregnancy would be fully, rather than partially informative.

## Current record of DNA-based prenatal diagnosis

The first use of RFLPs in prospective prenatal diagnosis of CF was reported by Farrall *et al.* (1986). Up to July 1987 some 70 couples in the United Kingdom with a 1 in 4 recurrence risk for CF had asked for first-trimester chorionic villus biopsy (M. Super, personal communication). Three had miscarried before biopsy and six shortly thereafter. In one case no CVS could be obtained, and in four cases the DNA yield was too low for analysis to be carried out. In the remaining pregnancies few difficulties were encountered in using the various probes for making diagnoses. Interestingly, three couples had asked for termination of pregnancy when the fetus was shown to have a 50 per cent risk of CF (see Fig. 5.3), while another couple in this situation had decided to continue the pregnancy. Amongst the 57 cases where a clear prediction could be made, 13 (23 per cent) had been deemed affected. At present there is no method of confirming the diagnosis of CF in a first-trimester abortus.

## Error rates in DNA-based diagnosis

In addition to the usual imperfections of laboratory testing (possibility of mix-up of samples, technical blemishes, erroneous interpretations), there is a source of error peculiar to the use of RFLPs in diagnosis. This is the possibility of recombination during meiosis between the marker and the gene being tracked. Recombination fractions are calculated from empirical data and are only as good as the effort which has been put into collecting large numbers of meioses, making sure that the families surveyed have genuine segregation of the appropriate disease, and ensuring that recombinants are not the results of non-paternity or non-maternity.

Estimates of the recombination fraction between the *D7S8* locus, defined by pJ3.11, and the *CF* locus suggest a figure of 0.003 (or 0.3 per cent), and between the *MET* locus and the *CF* locus a figure of 0.004 (0.4 per cent) (Beaudet *et al.* 1986). This means that there will be crossing-over or recombination in less than five out of every 1000 meioses. Preliminary data for *D7S23*, defined by probes pXV-2c and pCS.7, shows even tighter linkage with the *CF* locus (Estivill *et al.* 1987*a*). However, the recombination fraction between *D7S18*, defined by probe p7C22, and *CF* is of the order of 2.5 per cent, and that between *D7S13*, defined by probe p79a, and *CF* around 8 per cent. In both the latter cases there is a considerably greater cross-over rate for female meioses than for male meioses (M. Farrall, pers. commun.).

Calculations of exact error rates as a result of recombination need probability theory and are quite complex. In all cases they depend on the diagnosis made and the information used in reaching the diagnosis. In the most usual situation of a nuclear family and an index affected child being used to establish the phase of the markers, diagnosis of an affected fetus will be associated with an error which is approximately four times the recombination fraction. Diagnosis of a homozygous normal fetus leads to an error which is the square of the recombination fraction—for the *D7S8* or *MET* markers a vanishingly small number. If the prediction is for a heterozygote fetus, the error will be either approximately twice or three times the recombination fraction. With the exception of the *D7S18* and *D7S13* loci, these error rates are within acceptable limits.

## Heterozygote detection

One of the usual consequences of RFLP-based prenatal diagnosis is that carrier status can be established for unaffected fetuses. This is illustrated in

Fig. 5.4, where two of the Southern blot patterns show the fetus to be a heterozygote. Families who have an affected child may ask for the carrier status of unaffected siblings to be ascertained. At present such information is only useful if it excludes heterozygosity, since there is no way of establishing carrier status in the mating partner if he or she comes from a family with no history of CF. The sibling of a CF homozygote has a risk of 1 in 150 of producing an affected child if he/she married a random member of the United Kingdom population (Fig. 5.2). If this sibling is shown to be a carrier by DNA analysis, the risk of producing an affected child only rises to 1 in 100.

Although there are no reliable methods for detecting heterozygosity in members of families where CF is not known to be segregating, DNA analysis can modify the risks upward and downward from the population average of 1 in 25. Farrall *et al.* (1987) have pointed out that the *T1* allele at the XV-2c locus and the *H2* allele at the CS.7 locus occur much more frequently in association with the *CF* gene than would be expected by chance, because of linkage disequilibrium or allelic association. A random person with neither of these alleles (homozygous *T1/H2*) has a risk of being a carrier of only roughly 1 in 300. However, since this allelic combination (haplotype) does not occur all that often in the homozygous state, it is probably premature to use this form of DNA typing to modify the risks of heterozygosity.

## Microvillar enzyme-based prenatal diagnosis

In 1983 Carbarns *et al.* reported that the activities of two peptidases, γ-glutamyltranspeptidase (GGTP) and aminopeptidase M (APM), were significantly depressed in second-trimester amniotic fluid supernatant in the presence of a CF fetus. The fact that two separate enzymes, whose common feature was localization on the luminal surface of microvillar membranes, were co-ordinately reduced, suggested that some disturbance of the physiology rather than the biochemistry of CF was being detected. Van Diggelen *et al.* (1983) then showed that the amniotic fluid disaccharidases, sucrase, lactase, maltase, and trehalase were also reduced in CF. Very low levels of disaccharidase activity had previously been noted in cases of intestinal and anal obstruction (Morin *et al.* 1980). This pointed to a generalized reduction of amniotic fluid microvillar enzyme activities in CF, and suggested that either a viscid intestinal mucus or an actual obstruction of meconium passage in the affected fetus might be responsible.

This was confirmed by analysis of the isoenzymes of alkaline phosphatase (ALP). There are at least three major isoenzymes of ALP, coded for by three distinct genetic loci (Mulivor *et al.* 1978): placental ALP, intestinal ALP, and the bone/liver/kidney (BLK) form. Intestinal ALP is synthesized predominantly in the gut, both in the fetus and in the adult, and is the major isoenzyme found in second-trimester amniotic fluids (Mulivor et al. 1979). Using differential amino acid inhibition, Brock (1983) showed that the intestinal form was preferentially depleted when the fetus had CF. Subsequent analysis of ALP isoenzymes with specific monoclonal antibodies confirmed this finding (Brock et al. 1984a).

These observations, together with the fact that a very high proportion of newborn CF infants can be diagnosed from characteristic abnormalities of meconium composition, suggest that the simplest explanation for low microvillar enzyme activities in affected amniotic fluids is that the CF fetus has difficulty passing meconium in the second trimester. Several investigators have shown that disaccharidases (Antonowicz et al. 1974), peptidases (Jalanko et al. 1983), and ALP (Miki et al. 1978) have high specific activities in fetal intestinal mucosa by the beginning of the second trimester. Maximal activity is found in the proximal jejunum, with a decline down the rest of the small intestine (Antonowicz et al. 1974). Even higher specific activities of disaccharidases are found in meconium (Antonowicz et al. 1977). However, meconium disaccharidase activities appear to be greatest in the distal colon and fall away in the proximal colon and ileum (Potier et al. 1984). One thus gains a picture in the normal fetus of mucosal cells being sloughed off from the villi of the small intestine and passing down into the colon with increasing impaction and consequent elevation of the specific activities of the constituent microvillar enzymes.

It thus seems probable that the passage of meconium into amniotic fluid is impaired in the CF fetus at a critical stage in the second trimester. The primary evidence for this comes from the depleted levels of enzymes in amniotic fluid that could only originate in fetal gut. Confirmatory evidence is to be found in the occasional observations of abnormal ultrasonar scans (Muller et al. 1984a; Papp et al. 1985), suggesting a meconium plug in the ileum or jejunum. As outlined below, pathological examination of the second-trimester CF fetus has now shown clear evidence of very abnormal meconium constitution.

## Measurement of microvillar enzymes

In contrast to DNA analysis, measurement of microvillar enzymes is simple, quick, and cheap. Chromogenic substrates are available for GGTP, APM, and ALP, while maltase activity can be monitored with $p$-nitrophenyl-$\alpha$-D-glucopyranoside (Brock et al. 1984b). It is thus possible to measure four different microvillar enzymes on 50 $\mu$l of amniotic fluid in less than an hour. Estimation of the isoenzymes of ALP with a monoclonal antibody-based immunoassay (Brock et al. 1984a), though aesthetically pleasing, takes 18 hours and does not give superior precision to that achieved by the one-hour enzymatic assay (Brock et al. 1985).

Because the microvillar enzyme assay is monitoring a subtle clinical

Prenatal diagnosis

abnormality in the fetus, resolution of normal from abnormal amniotic fluid levels must be achieved empirically. The normal range is constructed from large numbers of amniotic fluids from unaffected pregnancies, and defined in terms of either percentiles or multiples of the median (Brock 1985). It is the practice in Edinburgh to use up to four enzymes in monitoring fetal CF, and to use a value equivalent to half the median at the relevant gestational week to define the cut-off. Obviously some cases of fetal CF will be above the cut-off (false negatives), while some normal fetuses will be below the cut-off (false positives). A typical spread of values is shown for the enzyme APM in Fig. 5.7.

The data for APM in Fig. 5.7 indicate the difficulties inherent in using indirect indicators of fetal CF to make judgements that may lead to

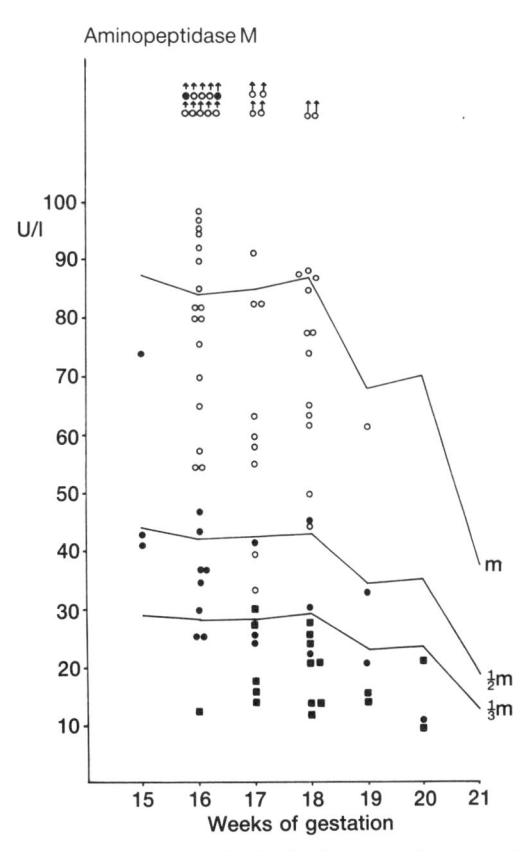

**Fig. 5.7.** APM activities in amniotic fluid. The normal range of values was constructed from 1000 samples and is defined in terms of a median (m) and fractions of the median. Individual values for pregnancies with 1 in 4 risk of CF are shown; ○, normal outcome; ●, affected outcome; ■, termination of pregnancy.

termination of pregnancy. Since mothers with an affected child have been reluctant to continue pregnancies where amniotic fluid microvillar enzyme values are abnormal, the validation of this system of diagnosis has rested to some extent on being able to confirm the predictions in the aborted fetus.

## Confirmation of diagnosis in the abortus

The clue to a method of diagnosing CF in the abortus came from the work of Muller *et al.* (1984*a*). They noted that when terminations of pregnancy were carried out in high-risk pregnancies with abnormal microvillar enzyme values, a substantial proportion of fetuses had a form of meconium ileus. In one case the intestinal abnormality was sufficiently pronounced to be visible on ultrasonar scan prior to termination. This was an unexpected finding in view of the fact that neonatal meconium ileus is usually only reported in some 7–10 per cent of CF infants. However, there seems no doubt that a majority of cases of fetal CF have grossly distended ileum and jejunum, filled with a green or black meconium with a sticky and glue-like consistency (Brock *et al.* 1985).

The abnormal meconium can be used as a biochemical basis for confirmation of diagnosis. In most fetuses thought to have CF, meconium albumin concentrations are enormously increased (Brock *et al.* 1985). However, as shown in Fig. 5.8 there are some albumins in the normal range. An interesting observation is that in these cases the trypsin-like protease levels are greatly increased. This led to the suggestion that there may have been a burst of pancreatic activity at some point between amniocentesis and termination of pregnancy, which could have degraded the more labile intestinal proteins. This hypothesis is supported by the finding of high concentrations of pancreatic oncofetal antigen in the meconium samples of fetuses with normal albumin and elevated proteases (Brock and Barron 1986). Pancreatic oncofetal antigen is synthesized mainly in the fetal pancreas, although it may also appear in the serum of adults with pancreatic carcinomas (Gelder *et al.* 1978).

Some doubts must remain about the validity of biochemical methods for confirmation of diagnosis of the CF fetus. Since amniotic fluid microvillar enzymes originate from the fetal gut, one would expect low values to be associated with disturbances in meconium passage, and to find an abnormal fetal meconium composition. If the pregnancy has a high risk of bearing a CF fetus, it can be assumed that in most cases the combination of low amniotic fluid microvillar enzymes and elevated meconium albumin or protease does indeed mean that the fetus has CF. However, there is a circularity in the argument that is uncomfortable.

The advent of RFLPs tightly linked to the *CF* gene has provided an independent method of verifying the diagnosis in an abortus. Curtis *et al.* (1988*a*) have shown that adequate amounts of undegraded DNA can be

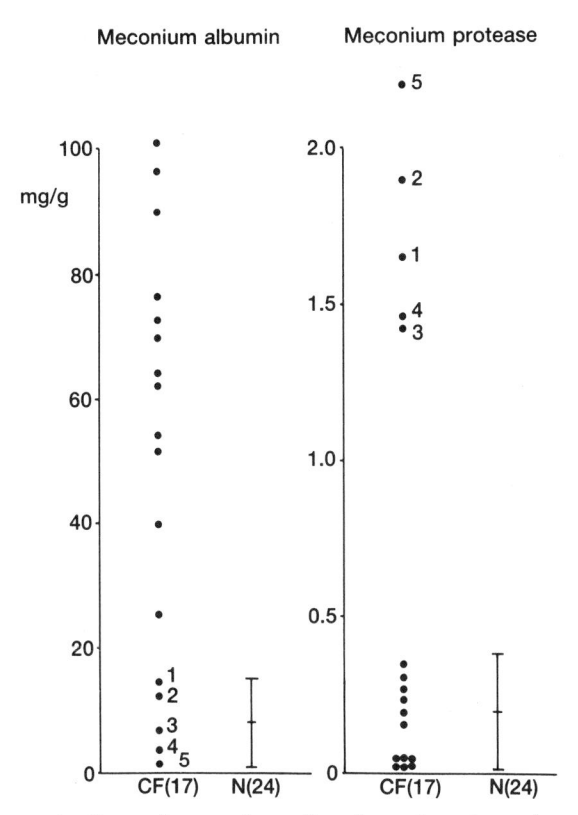

**Fig. 5.8.** Concentrations of meconium albumin and protease in samples from fetuses thought to have CF and from normal controls.

extracted from fetal intestine and other tissues, some of the samples having been stored frozen for up to three years. Obviously, tissues or cell lines from an index affected CF child are needed to establish the linkage phase of the DNA markers and to indicate the genotype expected in the fetal tissues. An example of this type of verification of diagnosis is shown in Fig. 5.9, where it can be seen that the essential information is provided by the pmet H and pmet D probes. Curtis *et al.* (1988a) typed eight abortuses, where termination of pregnancy had followed abnormal microvillar enzyme values, and found all eight to be confirmed by DNA analysis.

Even when there is no index affected child to establish phase, there is merit in genotyping the tissues of an abortus with DNA markers. In this instance the typing is used to establish phase for a subsequent first-trimester prenatal diagnosis, should it be needed. The assumption has to be made that the microvillar enzyme analysis had correctly identified a homozygous affected fetus, and that it is not a false positive. If it is a false positive (and these do

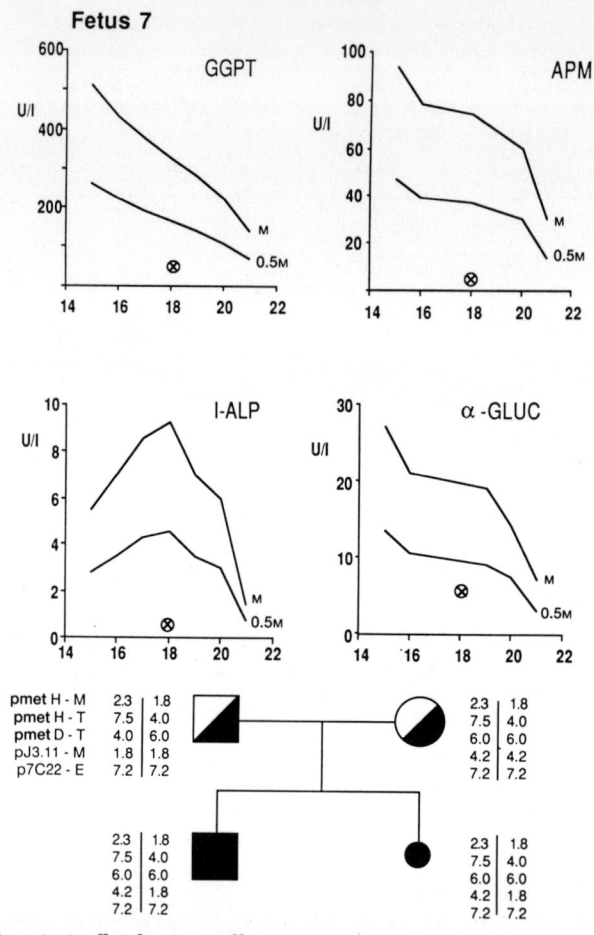

**Fig. 5.9.** Amniotic fluid microvillar enzyme activities in a sample where the fetus was diagnosed as having CF (upper part of figure). Pedigree and genotype of fetus, confirming the diagnosis as affected (lower part of figure).

occur—see below), the presumed relationship of the *CF* gene and the DNA markers will be wrong. However, it can be shown that in only about half of the subsequent prenatal diagnoses (i.e. half of the false positive rate) will a DNA-based diagnosis be incorrect, and in only a quarter will there be a missed case of CF. Thus, even if the false positive rate of microvillar enzyme testing is set as high as 10 per cent, only 2.5 per cent of subsequent DNA-based prenatal diagnosis will be false negatives.

# Current status of microvillar testing

## Optimal gestation

Most second-trimester amniocenteses are carried out at 16 weeks of gestation. Muller *et al.* (1984*b*) observed one pregnancy at risk for CF where marginally abnormal microvillar enzyme values at 16 weeks became clearly abnormal after a second amniocentesis at 18 weeks. Boué and Brock (1985) summarized their joint experience on microvillar testing, and concluded that false negative diagnosis could be reduced by carrying out analyses at 17 or 18 completed weeks of pregnancy. It is suggested that this narrow 'diagnostic window' should be checked by careful ultrasonar screening (Muller *et al.* 1985), and that the biparietal diameter should be between 38 and 44 mm (Boué *et al.* 1986).

## Enzyme analysis

Of the various microvillar enzymes which can be tested in amniotic fluid, most experience has been gained with GGTP, APM, intestinal ALP, and various disaccharidases. Measurement of disaccharidase activities is inconvenient, since amniotic fluid contains high concentrations of endogenous disaccharidases which must be removed by dialysis. The artificial substrate, $p$-nitrophenyl-$\alpha$-D-glucopyranoside, can be used to measure maltase activity without dialysis but, in the author's experience, gives a high false positive rate. The two laboratories with the largest prospective series (Edinburgh and Paris) rely on GGTP, APM, and ALP isoenzyme analysis.

Boué *et al.* (1986) reported 200 prospective diagnoses on pregnancies with a 1 in 4 risk of CF referred to their Paris centre. A large majority were on French couples who had ultrasonar scanning and amniocentesis carried out under tightly controlled conditions in just two hospitals. There was one case incorrectly predicted as abnormal amongst 142 normal infants (admitted false positive rate 0.7 per cent), and two missed cases of CF amongst 58 where the diagnosis was an affected fetus (admitted false negative rate 3.4 per cent). These are impressive figures. However, much depends on whether all of the 53 terminations of pregnancy were indeed CF. Of the 43 abortuses examined, all had the biochemical or macroscopic appearance of CF discussed on p. 3. Nonetheless, in this series there were apparently 58/200 (29.0 per cent) affected cases, more than expected in a Mendelian recessive condition. Boué *et al.* (1986) point out that when the index affected child had meconium ileus the recurrence rate was 47.2 per cent (25/53), whereas when the index affected child did not have meconium ileus the recurrence rate was 22.5 per cent (33/147). It is difficult to find any explanation for this extraordinary finding, and the suspicion remains that there were a number of unrecognized false positives. In fact, a false positive rate of 7 per cent would account for the excess of positives in the whole series.

A feature of the study by Boué *et al.* (1986) was the concordance between different microvillar enzymes in signalling a normal or affected pregnancy. Brock and Clarke (1987) have reported that occasionally GGTP behaves anomalously, and that very low GGTP values can be associated with normal APM and intestinal ALP values. In seven such pregnancies there were six liveborn outcomes with CF, and this pattern of activity must therefore be treated with suspicion. Brock *et al.* (1988) reported their own series of 258 pregnancies with a 1 in 4 risk of CF, and observed a false negative rate of 4.4 per cent and a false positive rate of 2.3 per cent. However, 32.2 per cent of the pregnancies in this series were found or predicted to be abnormal, suggesting a false positive rate of around 10 per cent.

## Predictability of microvillar testing

'Predictability' is a technical term indicating the proportion of cases where a diagnostic prediction is correct. It is usually expressed separately for positive (i.e. affected) and negative (i.e. unaffected) diagnoses, and can be formulated as an odds ratio or as a percentage. Predictabilities require an estimate of both false positive and false negative rates, and also knowledge of the prior odds in a pregnancy.

Predictabilities for microvillar testing on pregnancies with a 1 in 4 risk of CF are shown in Table 5.2. A range of false positive and false negative rates are given, and predictabilities are expressed both as odds and as percentages. It can be seen that the reliability is better for a normal test than for an abnormal one, since pregnancies start with the odds in favour of normality.

When predictabilities are calculated for pregnancies with lower prior odds of an affected fetus, the chances of a positive test signalling an affected fetus drop below 50 per cent. In Table 5.3 a false positive rate of 5 per cent and a false negative rate of 5 per cent are applied to the types of pregnancies shown in Fig. 5.2. In these cases the finding of abnormal microvillar enzyme values creates a predicament, since the chances are still weighted to normality in the fetus. For this reason microvillar enzyme testing should be used with caution on the low-risk pregnancy, and primarily serves the purpose of psychological reassurance.

**Table 5.2.** Predictabilities of microvillar enzyme testing in pregnancies with 1 in 4 prior odds

| False positive rate (%) | False negative rate (%) | Predictabilities Abnormal test | Normal test |
|---|---|---|---|
| 2 | 2 | 16.3 : 1 (94%) | 1 : 147 (0.7%) |
| 5 | 2 | 6.5 : 1 (87%) | 1 : 143 (0.7%) |
| 5 | 5 | 6.3 : 1 (86%) | 1 : 57 (1.7%) |
| 10 | 5 | 3.2 : 1 (76%) | 1 : 54 (1.9%) |

Table 5.3. Predictability of microvillar testing* for lower-risk pregnancies

| Prior odds | Predictabilities | |
|---|---|---|
| | Abnormal test | Normal test |
| 1 in 50  | 1 : 2.6 (28%)  | 1 : 951 (0.1%)   |
| 1 in 100 | 1 : 5.2 (16%)  | 1 : 1881 (0.05%) |
| 1 in 150 | 1 : 7.8 (11%)  | 1 : 2831 (0.04%) |
| 1 in 200 | 1 : 10.5 (9%)  | 1 : 3781 (0.03%) |

* Assuming a sensitivity of 95% and a specificity of 95%.

## Combining DNA and microvillar-based diagnosis

There are three general situations which are likely to be encountered when assessing a pregnancy with a 1 in 4 risk of CF. Each is likely to be handled in a slightly different way.

1. The nuclear family (father, mother, index affected child) is fully informative for one or more of the DNA probes (Table 5.1) in current usage, and the family present early enough in pregnancy for complete workup to be achieved. A first-trimester CVS will allow a firm diagnosis to be made. If the fetus is shown to be affected, there are great advantages in carrying out a termination of pregnancy at this early stage. If the fetus is unaffected, the temptation to confirm normality by second-trimester amniocentesis and microvillar enzyme assay should be resisted. The error rates associated with microvillar testing are sufficiently great to cause confusion and uncertainty if 'confirmatory' diagnosis is at variance with the primary diagnosis.

2. DNA probes cannot be used. The index affected child may have died before genotyping was possible. Both parents may be homozygous for all DNA probes available. The family may present too late for adequate workup to be completed. In these situations the method of choice is a second-trimester amniocentesis and microvillar enzyme assay.

3. The nuclear family is partially informative for available DNA probes. Here, careful counselling is called for. As shown in Fig. 5.3, there is a 50 per cent chance of excluding an affected fetus, and a 50 per cent chance of no diagnosis. In the latter situation the mother may opt for second-trimester amniocentesis, but even if the microvillar test signals normality there will be a residual risk of an affected fetus. By a curious mathematical quirk, because this mother starts with a higher risk of an affected fetus than the conventional 25 per cent, her posterior risk is still 5 per cent at a sensitivity and specificity of 95 per cent (Brock 1986). This is considerably greater than the 1.7 per cent

in Table 5.2. Mothers who have undergone both first-trimester CVS and second-trimester amniocentesis, and have still been left with a 5 per cent risk of bearing a child with CF, may feel that this is inadequate reassurance. The options open to partially informative couples should be spelled out before any procedures are undertaken.

## Summary

Two different methods of prenatal diagnosis of CF are currently available. Both are best suited to couples with a 1 in 4 risk of bearing an affected child, and should be applied with caution to lower-risk pregnancies.

The method of choice is first-trimester diagnosis on a CVS using linked DNA probes. The advantages are:

(1) the very high degree of accuracy of diagnosis; and
(2) the opportunity of first-trimester termination of pregnancy when the fetus is affected.

The disadvantages are:

(1) the need for a blood sample from an index affected child to establish phase;
(2) the requirement for early workup of the nuclear family to ascertain informativeness; and
(3) the chance that some families will be uninformative or only partially informative for available DNA probes.

An alternative form of diagnosis is that using microvillar enzyme testing on second-trimester amniocentesis samples. The advantages are:

(1) it is suitable for all pregnancies with a 1 in 4 risk of CF;
(2) no prior workup of the family is required; and
(3) assays can be completed within one hour of receipt of the sample.

The disadvantages are:

(1) the accuracy of diagnosis leaves scope for error; and
(2) if termination of pregnancy is indicated, this can only be carried out at about 18 or 19 weeks of pregnancy.

## Addendum

Since the main part of this review was written there have been several significant developments in the prenatal diagnosis of CF. The most important of these has been the ready availability of two probes at the *D7S23* locus, now thought to be within 'several tens of kilobases' of the *CF* locus, but not itself the *CF* locus (Farrall *et al.* 1988). One of these probes, pXV-2c, is described in Table 5.1, while the newer pKM.19 used with *Pst*I recognizes bands at 7.8 and 6.6 kbp, with a major allele frequency of 0.7 (Estivill *et al.* 1987*b*). The *D7S23* locus is now known to be on the centromeric side of the *CF* locus while the *D7S8* locus is towards the telomere (Farrall *et al.* 1988). Thus the probes pJ3.11 and the combination pKM.19/pXV-2c constitute flanking markers. However, the theoretical advantages of being able to use flanking markers to reduce diagnostic errors in prenatal diagnosis is not as great as it might be, given the 0.001 recombination fraction between *D7S23* and *CF* (Farrall *et al.* 1988) and the 0.003 recombination fraction between *D7S8* and *CF*.

With this battery of linked markers spanning the *CF* locus, it is most unusual to find a family where even one parent is homozygous for all the RFLPs (Weber *et al.* 1988). Up to January 1989, 191 prenatal diagnoses had been carried out on couples with a 1 in 4 risk of CF using linked DNA probes. Of these only 16 had been on half-informative pregnancies, and all were before the advent of *D7S23* probes. There were 3 cases where CVS failed and 11 miscarriages after the procedure. There were 2 false negatives, one thought to be the result of a cross-over between the *CF* and *MET* loci, and the other the consequence of typing fetal tissues after a false positive microvillar enzyme test. The proportion of cases predicted to be abnormal was not significantly different from Mendelian proportions (M. Super, personal communication).

There remains the continuing problem of providing prenatal diagnosis for couples whose affected child has already died. If a DNA sample from the child had been stored, or if fibroblasts have been cultured and preserved in frozen suspension, these may be recovered and used to establish the linkage phase of the markers (Curtis *et al.* 1988*b*). Of greater significance had been the observation that blood spots taken in the neonatal period for the Guthrie phenylketonuria test can be used to gain information on the marker genotype of a long-deceased CF child. The minute quantity of DNA in these blood spots is insufficient for conventional Southern blotting. However, specific base sequences can be amplified by a factor of $10^7$ to $10^9$ using the polymerase chain reaction (Saiki *et al.* 1988). Sequences surrounding the pKM.19/*Pst*I, the pCS7/*Hha*I, and the pJ3.11/*Pst*I polymorphic sites have been published (Feldman *et al.* 1988; Williams *et al.* 1988; Northrup *et al.* 1989), and several first-trimester prenatal diagnoses reported where the only information on the genotype of the deceased affected child came from a Guthrie blood-spot (Feldman *et al.* 1988; McIntosh *et al.* 1988).

Earlier reports of linkage disequilibrium between markers at the *D7S23* locus and the *CF* gene (Estivill *et al.* 1987*a*; Farrall *et al.* 1987) have been amply confirmed. The two systems on which most data have been accumulated are the pKM.19/*Pst*I and the pXV-2c/*Taq*I polymorphisms. The haplotype defined by the 7.8-kbp band at the former and the 2.1-kbp band at the latter, and usually known as *B*, is associated with the *CF* gene in 80 to 85 per cent of cases. In fact the frequency of the haplotype *B*/*CF* gene association in different north-European populations is remarkable; 0.81 for a British/Danish/Finnish mixture (Estivill *et al*, 1987*b*), 0.85 or 0.84 for Germans (Krawczak *et al*. 1988; Weber *et al*. 1988), 0.82 for Dutch (Te Meerman *et al*. 1988), and 0.80 for Scots (Curtis, personal communication). The frequency is slightly lower (0.73) amongst Italians and Spanish (Estivill *et al*. 1988), but was found to be 0.80 in a mixed group of North-American caucasians (Beaudet *et al*. 1986).

There have been various suggestions as to how linkage disequilibrium might be exploited in prenatal diagnosis of CF. Te Meerman *et al*. (1988) claimed that for a couple with a 1 in 4 risk of CF, but no affected child available for typing, some parental haplotype combinations could give predictive results where the final odds were comparable to those of microvillar enzyme testing. This was disputed by Holloway and Brock (1989), who calculated all the fetal risks associated with the 45 different parental combinations of *pXV-2c/pKM.19* haplotypes, using typical north-European linkage disequilibrium data. They found that in every case where the phase relationships of the two markers was unknown, at least one fetal genotype was associated with an intermediate risk of CF (Brock and Holloway, 1989). For example, if each parent is heterozygous for the pKM.19/*Pst*I and pXV-2c/*Taq*I polymorphisms, there are 9 different fetal genotypes possible with risks of 0.1, 0.8, 1.4, 2.3, 14.6, 37.4, 38.1, 60.4, and 95.6 per cent of being homozygous for the *CF* gene. The first four of these and the ninth are quite comparable to microvillar enzyme testing (1.7 or 80 per cent), but the others are too ambiguous to be useful. Obviously, a couple would not know in advance what fetal genotype would be found.

There is one area of prenatal diagnosis where linkage disequilibrium data has had practical usefulness. In a pregnancy with a 1 in 4 risk of CF, an abnormal microvillar enzyme test in the second trimester predicts affected status with a probability of about 80 per cent (see Table 5.2 and assume 8 per cent false positive rate and 5 per cent false negative rate.) Most parents opt for termination of such pregnancies. If they then seek a first-trimester prenatal diagnosis in a subsequent pregnancy, there is a temptation to use the tissues of the abortus to establish the linkage phase of the DNA markers. It was pointed out earlier that this would occasionally lead to both false positive and false negative diagnoses. However, if the tissues of the abortus are typed with pKM.19 and pXV-2c, a *BB* genotype will raise the probability of CF from 80 to over 95 per cent (Strain *et al*. 1988). All other fetal genotypes will lower the probability of CF. Thus for *BB* genotypes alone it is legitimate to use fetal tissues to establish the linkage phase of the markers.

# References

Antonowicz, I., Chang, S. K., and Grand, R. J. (1974). Development and distribution of lysosomal enzymes and disaccharidases in human fetal intestine. *Gastroenterology* **67**, 51–8.

Antonowicz, I., Milunsky, A., Lebenthal, E., and Shwachman, H. (1977). Disaccharidase and lysosomal enzyme activities in amniotic fluid, intestinal mucosa and meconium. *Biology of the Neonate* **32**, 280–9.

Beaudet, A. et al. (1986). Linkage of cystic fibrosis to two tightly linked DNA markers: joint report from a collaborative study. *American Journal of Human Genetics* **39**, 681–93.

Boué, A. and Brock, D. J. H. (1985). Prenatal diagnosis of cystic fibrosis. *Lancet* **i**, 47–8.

Boué, A. et al. (1986). Prenatal diagnosis in 200 pregnancies with a 1-in-4 risk of cystic fibrosis. *Human Genetics* **74**, 288–97.

Brock, D. J. H. (1983). Amniotic fluid alkaline phosphatase isoenzymes in early prenatal diagnosis of cystic fibrosis. *Lancet* **ii**, 941–43.

Brock, D. J. H. (1985). A comparative study of microvillar enzyme activities in the prenatal diagnosis of cystic fibrosis. *Prenatal Diagnosis* **5**, 129–34.

Brock, D. J. H. (1986). DNA probes or microvillar enzymes or both for prenatal diagnosis of cystic fibrosis. *Journal of Medical Genetics* **23**, 376–7.

Brock, D. J. H. and Barron, L. (1986). Biochemical analysis of meconium in fetuses presumed to have cystic fibrosis. *Prenatal Diagnosis* **6**, 291–8.

Brock, D. J. H. and Clarke, H. A. K. (1987). An abnormal pattern of amniotic fluid microvillar enzymes signalling fetal cystic fibrosis. *Clinical Genetics* **31**, 182–5.

Brock, D. J. H. and Holloway, S. H. (1989). Prenatal diagnosis of cystic fibrosis. *Lancet*, in press.

Brock, D. J. H., Bedgood, D., and Hayward, C. (1984a). Prenatal diagnosis of cystic fibrosis by assay of amniotic fluid microvillar enzymes. *Human Genetics* **65**, 248–51.

Brock, D. J. H., Barron, L., Bedgood, D. and Heyningen, V. van (1984b). Prenatal diagnosis of cystic fibrosis using a monoclonal antibody specific for intestinal alkaline phosphatase. *Prenatal Diagnosis* **4**, 421–6.

Brock, D. J. H., Bedgood, D., Barron, L., and Hayward, C. (1985). Prospective prenatal diagnosis of cystic fibrosis. *Lancet* **i**, 1175–8.

Brock, D. J. H., Clarke, H. A. K., and Barron, L. (1988). Prenatal diagnosis of cystic fibrosis by microvillar enzyme assay on a sequence of 258 pregnancies. *Human Genetics* **78**, 271–5.

Carbarns, N. J. B., Gosden, C., and Brock, D. J. H. (1983). Microvillar peptidase activity in amniotic fluid: possible use in the prenatal diagnosis of cystic fibrosis. *Lancet* **i**, 329–31.

Curtis, A., Strain, L., Mennie, M., and Brock, D. J. H. (1988a). Confirmation of prenatal diagnosis of cystic fibrosis by DNA typing of fetal tissues. *Journal of Medical Genetics* **25**, 79–82.

Curtis, A. et al. (1988b). First-trimester prenatal diagnosis of cystic fibrosis using fibroblasts from a deceased index child to establish haplotypes. *Prenatal Diagnosis* **8**, 625–8.

Diggelen, O.P. van, Janse, H.C., and Kleijer, W.J. (1983). Disaccharidases in amniotic fluid as possible prenatal marker for cystic fibrosis. *Lancet* **i**, 817.

Estivill, X., Schmidtke, J., Williamson, R., and Wainwright, B. (1986). Chromosome assignment and restriction fragment length polymorphism analysis of the anonymous DNA probe B79a at 7q22 (HMG8 assignment D7S13). *Human Genetics* **462**, 1-3.

Estivill, X. *et al.* (1987*a*). A candidate for the cystic fibrosis locus isolated by selection for methylation-free islands. *Nature* **326**, 840-5.

Estivill, X. *et al.* (1987*b*). Patterns of polymorphism and linkage disequilibrium for cystic fibrosis. *Genomics* **1**, 257-63.

Estivill, X. *et al.* (1988). Linkage disequilibrium between cystic fibrosis and linked DNA polymorphisms in Italian families: a collaborative study. *American Journal of Human Genetics* **43**, 23-28.

Farrall, M. *et al.* (1986). First-trimester prenatal diagnosis of cystic fibrosis with linked DNA probes. *Lancet* **i**, 1402-5.

Farrall, M., Estivill, X., and Williamson, R. (1987). Indirect cystic fibrosis carrier detection. *Lancet* **ii** 156-7.

Farrall, M. *et al.* (1988). Recombinations between *IRP* and cystic fibrosis. *American Journal of Human Genetics* **43**, 471-5.

Feldman, G.J., Williamson R., Beaudet, A.L., and O'Brien, W.E. (1988). Prenatal diagnosis of cystic fibrosis by DNA amplification for detection of KM-19 polymorphism. *Lancet* **ii**, 102.

Gelder, F.B., Reese, C.J., Moossa, A.R., Hall, T., and Hunter, R. (1978). Purification, partial characterization, and clinical evaluation of a pancreatic oncofetal antigen. *Cancer Research* **38**, 313-24.

Holloway, S.H. and Brock, D.J.H. (1989). Risks of fetal cystic fibrosis based on linkage disequilibrium data. *Human Genetics*, in press.

Jalanko, H., Ranta, T., Lehtonen, E., and Ruoslahti, E. (1983). $\gamma$-Glutamyl transpeptidase in human amniotic fluid and fetal tissues. *Clinica Chimica Acta* **134**, 337-46.

Kidd, V.J., Wallace, R.B., Itakura, K., and Woo, S.LC. (1983). $\alpha_1$-Antitrypsin deficiency detection by direct analysis of the mutation in the gene. *Nature* **304**, 230-4.

Knowlton, R.G., *et al.* (1985). A polymorphic DNA marker linked to cystic fibrosis is located on chromosome 7. *Nature* **318**, 380-5.

Krawczak, M. *et al* (1988). Allelic association of the cystic fibrosis locus and two DNA markers, XV2c and KM19, in 55 German families. *Human Genetics* **80**, 78-80.

McIntosh, I., Strain, L., and Brock, D.J.H. (1988). Prenatal diagnosis of cystic fibrosis where single affected child has died: Guthrie spots and microvillar enzyme testing. *Lancet* **ii**, 185.

Miki, K. *et al.* (1978). Human fetal organ alkaline phosphatase. *Clinica Chimica Acta* **85**, 115-24.

Morin, P.R., Potier, M., Dallaire, L., Melancon, S.B., and Milunsky, A. (1980). Prenatal detection of intestinal obstruction: deficient amniotic fluid disaccharidases in affected fetuses. *Clinical Genetics* **18**, 217-22.

Mulivor, R.A., Plotkin, L.I., and Harris, H. (1978). Differential inhibition of the

products of the human alkaline phosphatase loci. *Annals of Human Genetics* **42**, 1-13.
Mulivor, R. A., Mennuti, M. T., and Harris, H. (1979). Origin of the alkaline phosphatases in amniotic fluid. *American Journal of Obstetrics and Gynecology* **135**, 77-81.
Muller, F., Berg, S., Frot, J. C., Boué, J., and Boué, A. (1984*a*). Alkaline phosphatase isoenzyme assays for prenatal diagnosis of cystic fibrosis. *Lancet* i, 572.
Muller, F., Frot, J. C., Aubry, M. C., Boué, J., and Boué, A. (1984*b*). Meconium ileus in cystic fibrosis fetuses. *Lancet* ii, 223.
Muller, F., Berg, S., Frot, J. C., Boué, J. and Boué, A. (1985). Prenatal diagnosis of cystic fibrosis, I. Prospective study of 51 pregnancies. *Prenatal Diagnosis* **5**, 97.
Northrup, H., Rosenbloom, C., O'Brien, W. E., and Beaudet, A. L. (1989). Additional polymorphism for D7S8 linked to cystic fibrosis including detection by DNA amplification. *Nucleic Acids Research*, in press.
Papp, Z., Toth, Z., Szabo, M., and Szeifert, G. T. (1985). Early prenatal diagnosis of cystic fibrosis by ultrasound. *Clinical Genetics* **28**, 356-8.
Potier, M., Morin, P.-R., Melancon, S. B., and Dallaire, L. (1984). Differential stabilities of fetal intestinal disaccharidases determine their relative amounts released into amniotic fluid. *Biology of the Neonate* **45**, 257-60.
Saiki, R. K. *et al.* (1988). Primer-directed enzymatic amplification of DNA with a thermostable DNA polymerase. *Science* **239**, 487-91.
Scambler, P. J. *et al.* (1986). Isolation of a further anonymous informative DNA sequence from chromosome seven closely linked to cystic fibrosis. *Nuclei Acids Research* **14**, 1951-6.
Southern, E. M. (1975). Detection of specific sequences among DNA fragments separated by gel electrophoresis. *Journal of Molecular Biology* **98**, 503-17.
Strain, L., Curtis, A., Mennie, M., Holloway, S., and Brock, D. J. H. (1988). Use of linkage disequilibrium data in prenatal diagnosis of cystic fibrosis. *Human Genetics* **80**, 75-7,
Te Meerman, G. J. *et al.* (1988). Prenatal diagnosis of cystic fibrosis where single affected child has died. *Lancet* i, 745.
Tsui, L.-C. *et al.* (1985). Cystic fibrosis locus defined by a genetically linked polymorphic DNA marker. *Science* **230**, 1054-7.
Weber, J. *et al.* (1988). Cystic fibrosis:typing 89 German families with linked DNA probes. *Human Genetics* **81**, 54-6.
White, R. *et al.* (1985). A closely linked genetic marker for cystic fibrosis. *Nature* **318**, 382-4.
Williams, C. *et al.* (1988). Same-day, first-trimester antenatal diagnosis for cystic fibrosis by gene amplification. *Lancet* ii, 102-3.
Wilson, J. T. *et al.* (1982). Use of restriction endonucleases for mapping the allele for β globin. *Proceedings of the National Academy of Sciences USA* **79**, 3628-31.

# Index

A23187 33
abdomen, *see* gastrointestinal tract
acetylcholine 29, 30
*N*-acetylcysteine 16
adenocarcinoma 34
adolescence 8
   *see also* puberty
airway epithelia, *see* lungs
alcohol 16
alkaline phosphatase 77-80, 83-4
amiloride 25, 37
aminoglycosides 19
aminopeptidase M 77-80, 84
amniotic fluid, *see* microvillar enzyme-based prenatal diagnosis
anthracene-9-carboxylate 33
antibodies, *see* bacterial infections *and also specific types of*
arthropathy 6
aspergillosis 19
*Aspergillus fumigatus* 5, 18
aspirin 16
asthma, *see* lungs
ATP, *see* cell membranes
azlocillin 19

bacterial infections 5, 18-19
Bishop-Koop procedure 16
bleeding complications 19
blood cells 34-5
bowels, *see* gastrointestinal tract
breathing, *see* lungs
bronchodilators 17-18

calcium 30-1
   *see also* cell-membrane ion transport
calmodulin 35-6
cAMP 27, 30
cancer 15, 34
*Candida albicans* 18

carbachol 29
carbenicillin 19
carbohydrates, *see* nutrition
cell lines, and molecular genetics 57-61
cell-membrane ion transport 24-37
cell membranes 24-7
CF, *see* cystic fibrosis
*CF* gene, probes for detecting 70-1
   *see also* DNA technology, prenatal diagnosis
*CFAG* gene 45-6
chloride ions, and epithelial transport 24-7
chloride membrane channels, *see* cell-membrane ion transport
chorionic villus sampling, *see* prenatal diagnosis
chromosome 7 57-8
   map 48-50
chromosome-mediated gene transfer 56-61
chromosomes, *see* DNA technology, genetics; *see also* prenatal diagnosis
cimetidine 17
ciprofloxacin 19
cloning, *CF* region 56-8
*COL1A2* 48
complement 44
corticosteroids 18-19
Cri-du-chat syndrome 43
cystic fibrosis
   in adolescence 8
   arthropathy 6
   basic concepts in ix, 1-2, 12-13
   clinical features 3-4
   diabetes 6
   diagnosis 7
   family problems with 7-8
   gastrointestinal complications 15-16
   genetics and 2, 41-64
   growth and 6
   health-care delivery 21-2

*in vitro* cellular studies 24-37
linkage analysis 70-7
liver 5-6, 16-17
lungs 4-5, 17-18
management of 12-23
nutrition 14-15
pancreas 4, 6, 13-14, 33-4, 46
pathogenesis 2-3
pioneering work in 1-2
prenatal diagnosis 66-91
prognosis 8-10
psychological problems 20-1
in transport processes 24-40
cystic fibrosis antigen 45-6


*D7S8* 48, 50-1, 53-61
death, possibility 7-8
  *see also* prognostics
depression 7-8
dexamethasone 13
dextrans 37
diabetes mellitus 6, 13-14
diagnostics, of cystic fibrosis 7, 65-86
3′, 5-dichlorodiphenylamine-2-
  carboxylic acid 28
diet, *see* nutrition
disease locus, genetic mapping 43-4
DNA-based prenatal diagnosis,
  reliability 75-6
  error and 76
  and microvillar-enzyme-based 85-6
DNA, and prenatal diagnosis 67-70
DNA probes, and *CF* gene 70-1
DNA technology 41-64
  cloning, *CF* region 56-61
  'jumping' libraries 53-6
  'linking' libraries 53-6
  PGFE 52-3
  recent 52-62


electrical processes, and sweating 28-9
enzyme-based prenatal diagnosis, *see*
  microvillar enzyme-based prenatal
  diagnosis
epithelial ion transport 24-40
exercise, and respiration, *see* lungs
exocrine glands 2-3
  *see also* sweat glands, salivary glands

family problems 7-8
family trees 42-4
fats, *see* nutrition
ferritin 15
fibroblasts 35
fibrosis, pancreatic, *see* pancreatic
  insufficiency
flucloxacillin 18
food, *see* nutrition
forkolin 33, 35
frusemide 25
fungal infections 19


gallstones 17
gastrografin 15
gastrointestinal tract 3-4, 15-16
  epithelia in 34
gene libraries, *see* DNA technology
gene mapping 41-65
  molecular 41-65
  prenatal diagnosis 65-91
genetics 2, 22, 41-64
  classical 42, 44-6
  prenatal diagnosis and 66-91
  reverse 42, 47-61
gentamicin 19
γ-glutamyltranspeptidase 77-80, 83-4
golytely 16
growth 6
  *see also* nutrition


haematemesis 16-17
haemophilia 44
*Haemophilus influenzae* 5, 18
haemoptysis 5
health-care delivery 21-2
heart-lung transplantation 20
heat 13
  *see also* sweat glands
hepatic failure, *see* liver
heterozygote detection 76-7
5-hydroxytryptamine 30


immunization 18
immunoreactive trypsin 7, 22
immunoreactive trypsin assay 7, 22
infection, *see* bacterial infections, viral
  infections

# Index

infertility, male 3, 21
insulin, 14
  see also diabetes mellitus, pancreas
intestinal obstruction 3-4
  see also gastrointestinal system
intussusception 16
  see also gastrointestinal tract
ion transport processes 24-40
iron-deficiency anaemia 15
isoprenaline 29, 31, 33-4

joint diseases 6
'jumping' libraries 53-6

$\beta$-lactam drugs 19
linked markers 49-50
  to the genes 50-1
  use of 48-50
'linking' libraries 53-6
liver 3, 5-6, 16-17
Lorist 6 60
lungs 3-5, 17-18, 30-3
  bleeding complications 19
  transplantation 20
  transport of ions, epithelial 30-3
  X-rays 5, 19
lymphocytes 34-5

malnutrition, see nutrition
mapping, of genes, see DNA
  technology, gene mapping; see also
  prenatal diagnosis
meconium ileus 4, 15-16
  equivalent 16
MET 48, 50, 53-61
microvillar enzyme-based prenatal
  diagnosis 77-85
  diagnosis, in abortus 80-3
  DNA based 85-6
  measurement and 78-80
  predictability of 84
  state-of-the-art 83-4
MNNG-HOS cell line 58-9
molecular genetics, see genetics
mRNA 36
mucopolysaccharidosis 44
'mucoviscidosis' 1
mucus, lungs, see bacterial infections

muscular dystrophy 43-4
mutagenized human osteosarcoma cell
  line, see MNNG-HOS

nasal obstruction 18
nasal polyps 18
neonatal screening 22
  see also prenatal diagnosis
netilmicin 19
neurotransmitters, see specific names of
norfloxacin 19
nutrition 6, 14-15

outlook, in cystic fibrosis, see
  prognostics

pancreas 2-4, 13-14, 33-4, 46
  and diabetes, see diabetes mellitus
pancreatic enzymes, see pancreatic
  insufficiency
pancreatic fibrosis, see pancreatic
  insufficiency
pancreatic insufficiency 4, 13-14, 46
pancreatin 13
paroxonase, see PON
patch clamping technique 32-3
pathogenesis, of cystic fibrosis 2-3
penicillin 19
PFGE 52-3
PIC value 47
piretanide 25
pitressin 16-17
pneumothorax 5
polymorphism information content, see
  PIC value
polyps, nasal 18
PON 47-8
potassium ions, and membranes 24-7
pregnancy 21
  informative, and cystic fibrosis 71-5
  see also prenatal diagnosis
prenatal diagnosis, of cystic
  fibrosis 66-91
  combined DNA/microvillar-
  based 85-6
  by linkage analysis 70-7
  microvillar enzyme-based 77-8
prognostics 8-10

prostaglandins 36
proteins, *see* nutrition
*Pseudomonas aeruginosa* 5, 18
*Pseudomonas cepacia* 18
psychiatric problems 7-8, 20-1
puberty 6, 8, 21
pulse field gel electrophoresis, *see* PFGE
pyrazine carboxamides 25

random markers, and *CF* gene 47
ranitidine 17
'rare cutter' enzymes 54-6
β-receptor activation 29-30
rectal prolapse 16
red cells 34-5
reverse genetics 42, 47-61
RFLPs 41, 43, 47-8, 69-71

salbutamol 17
salivary glands 33-4
salt (sodium chloride), *see* sweat glands
segregation analysis, genes 43-8
  linking *CF* gene with random markers 47
  mapping disease locus 43-4
selenium 15
social problems, and cystic fibrosis 7-8, 20-1
sodium bicarbonate 13
sodium chloride 24-7
  *see also* sweat glands
Southern blot analysis 72-5
sputum, blood in 19
*Staphylococcus aureus* 5, 18

steatorrhoea, *see* pancreatic insufficiency
surgery, and bowel 15-16
survival, in cystic fibrosis, *see* prognostics, in cystic fibrosis
SV40-mediated cellular transformation 57-8
sweat, composition of 27
sweat glands 3, 7, 13, 27
  electrical processes 28-9
sweat tests 7
sweating rate 28

*TCRB* 48
testes 3, 21
tobramycin 19
trace elements 15
transepithelial ion transport 24-40
trypsin 7, 22
tumor cell lines, and gene mapping 57-61

vasoactive intestinal polypeptide (VIP) 30, 34
viral infections 5
vitamin K, *see* nutrition
vitamins, *see* nutrition
volvulus 15
  *see also* gastrointestinal system

*Xenopus* 36
xeroderma pigmentosum 44
X-rays, of lungs 5, 19

zinc 15